ADA is the official and definit

CDT®
2021

Current
Dental
Terminology

Includes app and e-book

ADA American Dental Association®
America's leading advocate for oral health

Book ISBN: 978-1-68447-059-4

E-book ISBN: 978-1-68447-060-0

ADA Product No.: J021BT

Acknowledgments

The American Dental Association's Council on Dental Benefit Programs, Practice Institute and Department of Product Development and Sales developed this publication.

Principal staff contributions were made by Dr. Krishna Aravamudhan, Sr. Director, Center for Dental Benefits, Coding & Quality; Frank Pokorny, MBA, FACD (hon.), Senior Manager, Dental Codes Maintenance and Development; Stacy Starnes, Dental Code Advisor; Pamela Woolf, Senior Manager Product Development; and Kathy Pulkrabek, Manager/Editor, Professional Products.

CDT 2021 Current Dental Terminology

Table of Contents

Preface

Introduction

This reference manual, published by the ADA, contains the *Code on Dental Procedures and Nomenclature* (CDT Code) version that is effective for services provided on or after January 1, 2021 through December 31, 2021.

In August 2000 the CDT Code was designated by the federal government as the national terminology for reporting dental services on claims submitted to third-party payers, in accordance with authority granted by the Health Insurance Portability and Accountability Act of 1996 (HIPAA).

The ADA's Council on Dental Benefit Programs is responsible for maintaining the CDT Code in accordance with ADA Bylaws and policy, and applicable federal regulations. *Current Dental Terminology (CDT)* technical content is developed by staff in the ADA Practice Institute's Center for Dental Benefits Coding and Quality, while responsibility for this manual's printing, pricing and distribution of falls to the ADA's Department of Product Development and Sales.

- **Should you have any recommendations for CDT Code additions, revisions or deletions**, direct access to the process is via the portal established at *ADA.org/cdt*.

- **For questions about dental procedure coding or claim submission** email *msc@ADA.org* or call the ADA Member Service Center at 800.947.4746. Support is available from 8:30 a.m. to 6:00 p.m. Central Time, Monday through Friday.

- **For general information about, or to pursue CDT Code licensing**, visit *ADA.org/CDTlicensing*. In addition to information about licensing this site contains the questionnaire that must be completed as the first step of the licensing process.

- **For any questions regarding pricing or purchasing additional copies of CDT** visit *ADAcatalog.org* or call 800.947.4746. If you are ordering 25 or more copies or if you are ordering for an educational institution, please email *SpecialOrdersPDS@ADA.org* to request a quote.

Categories of Service

The CDT Code is organized into twelve categories of service, each with its own series of five-digit alphanumeric codes:

Category of Service	Code Series
I. Diagnostic	D0100–D0999
II. Preventive	D1000–D1999
III. Restorative	D2000–D2999
IV. Endodontics	D3000–D3999
V. Periodontics	D4000–D4999
VI. Prosthodontics, removable	D5000–D5899
VII. Maxillofacial Prosthetics	D5900–D5999
VIII. Implant Services	D6000–D6199
IX. Prosthodontics, fixed	D6200–D6999
X. Oral & Maxillofacial Surgery	D7000–D7999
XI. Orthodontics	D8000–D8999
XII. Adjunctive General Services	D9000–D9999

These categories exist solely as a means to organize the CDT Code. As a result, some categories of service are divided into subcategories of related procedures. Many categories and subcategories have descriptors applicable to all procedure codes therein.

Dental procedure codes within a Category of Service, or a subcategory, are not always listed in numeric order. The reason is that existing numeric sequences often do not have unassigned codes available for CDT Code additions.

Such out of sequence listings are in the following Categories of Service (or subcategories therein): Diagnostic; Restorative; Periodontics; Maxillofacial Prosthetics; Implant Services; Oral & Maxillofacial Surgery; Adjunctive General Services.

Preface

Components of a Dental Procedure Code Entry

Every procedure in the CDT Code must have the first two of the following three components:

1. Procedure Code

A five character alphanumeric code beginning with the letter "D" that identifies a specific dental procedure. A Procedure Code cannot be changed or abbreviated.

2. Nomenclature

The written title of a Procedure Code. Nomenclature may be abbreviated when printed on claim forms or other documents that are subject to space limitation. Any such abbreviation does not constitute a change to the Nomenclature.

3. Descriptor

A written narrative that further defines the nature and intended use of a single Procedure Code, or group of such codes. A Descriptor, when present, follows the applicable Procedure Code and its Nomenclature. Descriptors that apply to a series of Procedure Codes precede that series of codes.

Using the CDT Code

The following points should prove helpful when using the CDT Code for recording services provided on the patient record, and when reporting procedures on a paper or electronic claim submission.

1. The presence of a CDT Code does not mean that the procedure is:
   a. endorsed by any entity or is considered a standard of care
   b. covered or reimbursed by a dental benefits plan

2. General practitioners, specialists, and other individuals may report any of the listed CDT Codes as long as they are delivering procedures and services within the scope of their state law.

3. CDT Codes that require inclusion of a narrative description on the claim have the words "by report" in their nomenclature.

4. "Unspecified... procedure, by report" codes are used when, in the opinion of the dentist, there is no other CDT Code entry that accurately describes the services provided to the patient.

5. Documentation of services provided may necessitate selection of CDT Codes from different categories of service. Two illustrative scenarios follow. Section 4 "Alphabetic Index to the CDT Code" (starting on page 139) will also help you locate the page number for an applicable procedure code.

Preface

Scenario Description	Procedure Delivered	Category of Service
1. Implant Case – Four-unit Fixed Partial Denture	Radiographs	Diagnostic D0100–D0999
	Implant body placement	Implant Services D6000–D6199
	Implant supported retainers	
	Pontics	Prosthodontics, fixed D6200–D6999
2. Orthodontic Case – Treatment Planning	Pre-treatment examination	Orthodontics D8000–D8999
	Radiographs	Diagnostic D0100–D0999
	Diagnostic casts	
	Case presentation	Adjunctive General Services D9000–D9999

Required Statement

If there is more than one code in this edition that consists of a procedure and a dentist submits a claim under one of these codes, the payor may process the claim under any of these codes that is consistent with the payor's reimbursement policy.

Section 1

Code on Dental Procedures and Nomenclature (CDT Code)

The current version of the *Code on Dental Procedures and Nomenclature* (CDT Code) that follows is effective for the calendar year 2021. There are a number of changes from the prior version, which are identified by the following symbols:

- ● New procedure code
- ▲ Substantive revision to a nomenclature or descriptor
- # Editorial

Dental procedure codes that are no longer valid are not present. Chapter 2 contains the summary of all additions, revisions and deletions effective January 1, 2021.

As noted in the "Preface" the CDT Code is divided into twelve Categories of Service.

Please note that when a code's nomenclature includes a "by report" notation, a narrative explaining the treatment provided must be included with the claim submission.

Classification of Materials

Names of dental materials are included in numerous procedure nomenclatures within several Categories of Service (e.g., Restorative; Prosthodontics, fixed; etc.). The following list of dental materials is included in the CDT Code **solely to aid selection** of a procedure code applicable to the service provided.

- **Classification of Metals** *(Source: ADA Council on Scientific Affairs)*
  The noble metal classification system has been adopted as a more precise method of reporting various alloys used in dentistry. The alloys are defined on the basis of the percentage of metal content.

Classification	Requirement
High Noble Alloys	Noble Metal Content ≥ 60% (gold+ platinum group*) and gold ≥ 40%
Titanium and Titanium Alloys	Titanium ≥ 85%
Noble Alloys	Noble Metal Content ≥ 25% (gold + platinum group*)
Predominantly Base Alloys	Noble Metal Content < 25% (gold + platinum group*)

* metals of the platinum group are platinum, palladium, rhodium, iridium, osmium and ruthenium

- **Porcelain/ceramic**
  Refers to pressed, fired, polished or milled materials containing predominantly inorganic refractory compounds including porcelains, glasses, ceramics, and glass-ceramics.

- **Resin**
  Refers to any resin-based composite, including fiber or ceramic reinforced polymer compounds, and glass ionomers.

D0100–D0999 I. Diagnostic

Clinical Oral Evaluations

The codes in this section recognize the cognitive skills necessary for patient evaluation. The collection and recording of some data and components of the dental examination may be delegated; however, the evaluation, which includes diagnosis and treatment planning, is the responsibility of the dentist. As with all ADA procedure codes, there is no distinction made between the evaluations provided by general practitioners and specialists. Report additional diagnostic or definitive procedures separately.

 # D0120 periodic oral evaluation – established patient
An evaluation performed on a patient of record to determine any changes in the patient's dental and medical health status since a previous comprehensive or periodic evaluation. This includes an oral cancer evaluation, periodontal screening where indicated, and may require interpretation of information acquired through additional diagnostic procedures. Report additional diagnostic procedures separately.

D0140 limited oral evaluation – problem focused
An evaluation limited to a specific oral health problem or complaint. This may require interpretation of information acquired through additional diagnostic procedures. Report additional diagnostic procedures separately. Definitive procedures may be required on the same date as the evaluation.

Typically, patients receiving this type of evaluation present with a specific problem and/or dental emergencies, trauma, acute infections, etc.

D0145 oral evaluation for a patient under three years of age and counseling with primary caregiver
Diagnostic services performed for a child under the age of three, preferably within the first six months of the eruption of the first primary tooth, including recording the oral and physical health history, evaluation of caries susceptibility, development of an appropriate preventive oral health regimen and communication with and counseling of the child's parent, legal guardian and/or primary caregiver.

 # D0150 comprehensive oral evaluation – new or established patient
Used by a general dentist and/or a specialist when evaluating a patient comprehensively. This applies to new patients; established patients who have had a significant change in health conditions or other unusual circumstances, by report, or established patients who have been absent from active treatment for three or more years. It is a thorough evaluation

and recording of the extraoral and intraoral hard and soft tissues. It may require interpretation of information acquired through additional diagnostic procedures. Additional diagnostic procedures should be reported separately.

This includes an evaluation for oral cancer, the evaluation and recording of the patient's dental and medical history and a general health assessment. It may include the evaluation and recording of dental caries, missing or unerupted teeth, restorations, existing prostheses, occlusal relationships, periodontal conditions (including periodontal screening and/or charting), hard and soft tissue anomalies, etc.

D0160 detailed and extensive oral evaluation – problem focused, by report
A detailed and extensive problem focused evaluation entails extensive diagnostic and cognitive modalities based on the findings of a comprehensive oral evaluation. Integration of more extensive diagnostic modalities to develop a treatment plan for a specific problem is required. The condition requiring this type of evaluation should be described and documented.

Examples of conditions requiring this type of evaluation may include dentofacial anomalies, complicated perio-prosthetic conditions, complex temporomandibular dysfunction, facial pain of unknown origin, conditions requiring multi-disciplinary consultation, etc.

D0170 re-evaluation – limited, problem focused (established patient; not post-operative visit)
Assessing the status of a previously existing condition. For example:
- a traumatic injury where no treatment was rendered but patient needs follow-up monitoring;
- evaluation for undiagnosed continuing pain;
- soft tissue lesion requiring follow-up evaluation.

D0171 re-evaluation – post-operative office visit

D0180 comprehensive periodontal evaluation – new or established patient
This procedure is indicated for patients showing signs or symptoms of periodontal disease and for patients with risk factors such as smoking or diabetes. It includes evaluation of periodontal conditions, probing and charting, evaluation and recording of the patient's dental and medical history and general health assessment. It may include the evaluation and recording of dental caries, missing or unerupted teeth, restorations, occlusal relationships and oral cancer evaluation.

     ● new procedure code   ▲ revision to a nomenclature or descriptor   # Editorial

Pre-diagnostic Services

D0190 **screening of a patient**
A screening, including state or federally mandated screenings, to determine an individual's need to be seen by a dentist for diagnosis.

D0191 **assessment of a patient**
A limited clinical inspection that is performed to identify possible signs of oral or systemic disease, malformation, or injury, and the potential need for referral for diagnosis and treatment.

Diagnostic Imaging

Should be taken only for clinical reasons as determined by the patient's dentist. Should be of diagnostic quality and properly identified and dated. Is a part of the patient's clinical record and the original images should be retained by the dentist. Originals should not be used to fulfill requests made by patients or third-parties for copies of records.

Image Capture with Interpretation

D0210 **intraoral – complete series of radiographic images**
A radiographic survey of the whole mouth, usually consisting of 14–22 periapical and posterior bitewing images intended to display the crowns and roots of all teeth, periapical areas and alveolar bone.

D0220 **intraoral – periapical first radiographic image**

D0230 **intraoral – periapical each additional radiographic image**

D0240 **intraoral – occlusal radiographic image**

D0250 **extra-oral – 2D projection radiographic image created using a stationary radiation source, and detector**
These images include, but are not limited to: Lateral Skull; Posterior-Anterior Skull; Submentovertex; Waters; Reverse Tomes; Oblique Mandibular Body; Lateral Ramus.

D0251 **extra-oral posterior dental radiographic image**
Image limited to exposure of complete posterior teeth in both dental arches. This is a unique image that is not derived from another image.

D0270 **bitewing – single radiographic image**

D0272 **bitewings – two radiographic images**

D0273 **bitewings – three radiographic images**

D0274 bitewings – four radiographic images

D0277 vertical bitewings – 7 to 8 radiographic images
This does not constitute a full mouth intraoral radiographic series.

D0310 sialography

D0320 temporomandibular joint arthrogram, including injection

D0321 other temporomandibular joint radiographic images, by report

D0322 tomographic survey

D0330 panoramic radiographic image

D0340 2D cephalometric radiographic image – acquisition, measurement and analysis
Image of the head made using a cephalostat to standardize anatomic positioning, and with reproducible x-ray beam geometry.

D0350 2D oral/facial photographic image obtained intra-orally or extra-orally

D0351 3D photographic image
This procedure is for dental or maxillofacial diagnostic purposes. Not applicable for a CAD-CAM procedure.

D0364 cone beam CT capture and interpretation with limited field of view – less than one whole jaw

D0365 cone beam CT capture and interpretation with field of view of one full dental arch – mandible

D0366 cone beam CT capture and interpretation with field of view of one full dental arch – maxilla, with or without cranium

D0367 cone beam CT capture and interpretation with field of view of both jaws; with or without cranium

D0368 cone beam CT capture and interpretation for TMJ series including two or more exposures

D0369 maxillofacial MRI capture and interpretation

D0370 maxillofacial ultrasound capture and interpretation

D0371 sialoendoscopy capture and interpretation

Image Capture Only

Capture by a Practitioner not associated with Interpretation and Report

D0380 **cone beam CT image capture with limited field of view – less than one whole jaw**

D0381 **cone beam CT image capture with field of view of one full dental arch – mandible**

D0382 **cone beam CT image capture with field of view of one full dental arch – maxilla, with or without cranium**

D0383 **cone beam CT image capture with field of view of both jaws, with or without cranium**

D0384 **cone beam CT image capture for TMJ series including two or more exposures**

D0385 **maxillofacial MRI image capture**

D0386 **maxillofacial ultrasound image capture**

- **D0701** **panoramic radiographic image – image capture only**

- **D0702** **2-D cephalometric radiographic image – image capture only**

- **D0703** **2-D oral/facial photographic image obtained intra-orally or extra-orally – image capture only**

- **D0704** **3-D photographic image – image capture only**

- **D0705** **extra-oral posterior dental radiographic image – image capture only**
  Image limited to exposure of complete posterior teeth in both dental arches. This is a unique image that is not derived from another image.

- **D0706** **intraoral – occlusal radiographic image – image capture only**

- **D0707** **intraoral – periapical radiographic image – image capture only**

- **D0708** **intraoral – bitewing radiographic image – image capture only**
  Image axis may be horizontal or vertical.

- **D0709** **intraoral – complete series of radiographic images – image capture only**
  A radiographic survey of the whole mouth, usually consisting of 14–22 images (periapical and posterior bitewing as indicated) intended to display the crowns and roots of all teeth, periapical areas and alveolar bone.

Interpretation and Report Only

Interpretation and Report by a Practitioner not associated with Image Capture

D0391 **intraoral – complete series of radiographic images – image capture only**

Post Processing of Image or Image Sets

D0393 **treatment simulation using 3D image volume**
The use of 3D image volumes for simulation of treatment including, but not limited to, dental implant placement, orthognathic surgery and orthodontic tooth movement.

D0394 **digital subtraction of two or more images or image volumes of the same modality**
To demonstrate changes that have occurred over time.

D0395 **fusion of two or more 3D image volumes of one or more modalities**

Tests and Examinations

D0411 **HbA1c in-office point of service testing**

D0412 **blood glucose level test – in-office using a glucose meter**
This procedure provides an immediate finding of a patient's blood glucose level at the time of sample collection for the point-of-service analysis.

D0414 **laboratory processing of microbial specimen to include culture and sensitivity studies, preparation and transmission of written report**

D0415 **collection of microorganisms for culture and sensitivity**

D0416 **viral culture**
A diagnostic test to identify viral organisms, most often herpes virus.

D0417 **collection and preparation of saliva sample for laboratory diagnostic testing**

D0418 **analysis of saliva sample**
Chemical or biological analysis of saliva sample for diagnostic purposes.

D0419 **assessment of salivary flow by measurement**
This procedure is for identification of low salivary flow in patients at risk for hyposalivation and xerostomia, as well as effectiveness of pharmacological agents used to stimulate saliva production.

D0422 **collection and preparation of genetic sample material for laboratory analysis and report**

D0423 **genetic test for susceptibility to diseases – specimen analysis**
Certified laboratory analysis to detect specific genetic variations associated with increased susceptibility for diseases.

D0425 **caries susceptibility tests**
Not to be used for carious dentin staining.

D0431 **adjunctive pre-diagnostic test that aids in detection of mucosal abnormalities including premalignant and malignant lesions, not to include cytology or biopsy procedures**

D0460 **pulp vitality tests**
Includes multiple teeth and contra lateral comparison(s), as indicated.

D0470 **diagnostic casts**
Also known as diagnostic models or study models.

D0600 **non-ionizing diagnostic procedure capable of quantifying, monitoring, and recording changes in structure of enamel, dentin, and cementum**

D0601 **caries risk assessment and documentation, with a finding of low risk**
Using recognized assessment tools.

D0602 **caries risk assessment and documentation, with a finding of moderate risk**
Using recognized assessment tools.

D0603 **caries risk assessment and documentation, with a finding of high risk**
Using recognized assessment tools.

- **D0604** **antigen testing for a public health related pathogen, including coronavirus**

- **D0605** **antibody testing for a public health related pathogen, including coronavirus**

Oral Pathology Laboratory

These procedures do not include collection of the tissue sample, which is documented separately.

D0472 **accession of tissue, gross examination, preparation and transmission of written report**
To be used in reporting architecturally intact tissue obtained by invasive means.

D0473 **accession of tissue, gross and microscopic examination, preparation and transmission of written report**
To be used in reporting architecturally intact tissue obtained by invasive means.

D0474 **accession of tissue, gross and microscopic examination, including assessment of surgical margins for presence of disease, preparation and transmission of written report**
To be used in reporting architecturally intact tissue obtained by invasive means.

D0480 **accession of exfoliative cytologic smears, microscopic examination, preparation and transmission of written report**
To be used in reporting disaggregated, non-transepithelial cell cytology sample via mild scraping of the oral mucosa.

D0486 **laboratory accession of transepithelial cytologic sample, microscopic examination, preparation and transmission of written report**
Analysis, and written report of findings, of cytological sample of disaggregated transepithelial cells.

D0475 **decalcification procedure**
Procedure in which hard tissue is processed in order to allow sectioning and subsequent microscopic examination.

D0476 **special stains for microorganisms**
Procedure in which additional stains are applied to biopsy or surgical specimen in order to identify microorganisms.

D0477 **special stains, not for microorganisms**
Procedure in which additional stains are applied to a biopsy or surgical specimen in order to identify such things as melanin, mucin, iron, glycogen, etc.

D0478 **immunohistochemical stains**
A procedure in which specific antibody based reagents are applied to tissue samples in order to facilitate diagnosis.

D0479 **tissue in–situ hybridization, including interpretation**
A procedure which allows for the identification of nucleic acids, DNA and RNA, in the tissue sample in order to aid in the diagnosis of microorganisms and tumors.

D0481 **electron microscopy**

D0482 **direct immunofluorescence**
A technique used to identify immunoreactants which are localized to the patient's skin or mucous membranes.

D0483 **indirect immunofluorescence**
A technique used to identify circulating immunoreactants.

D0484 **consultation on slides prepared elsewhere**
A service provided in which microscopic slides of a biopsy specimen prepared at another laboratory are evaluated to aid in the diagnosis of a difficult case or to offer a consultative opinion at the patient's request. The findings are delivered by written report.

D0485 **consultation, including preparation of slides from biopsy material supplied by referring source**
A service that requires the consulting pathologist to prepare the slides as well as render a written report. The slides are evaluated to aid in the diagnosis of a difficult case or to offer a consultative opinion at the patient's request.

D0502 **other oral pathology procedures, by report**

D0999 **unspecified diagnostic procedure, by report**
Used for a procedure that is not adequately described by a code. Describe the procedure.

D1000–D1999 II. Preventive

Dental Prophylaxis

▲ **D1110** **prophylaxis – adult**
Removal of plaque, calculus and stains from the tooth structures and implants in the permanent and transitional dentition. It is intended to control local irritational factors.

▲ **D1120** **prophylaxis – child**
Removal of plaque, calculus and stains from the tooth structures and implants in the primary and transitional dentition. It is intended to control local irritational factors.

Topical Fluoride Treatment (Office Procedure)

Prescription strength fluoride product designed solely for use in the dental office, delivered to the dentition under the direct supervision of a dental professional. Fluoride must be applied separately from prophylaxis paste.

D1206 **topical application of fluoride varnish**

D1208 **topical application of fluoride – excluding varnish**

Other Preventive Services

D1310 **nutritional counseling for control of dental disease**
Counseling on food selection and dietary habits as a part of treatment and control of periodontal disease and caries.

D1320 **tobacco counseling for the control and prevention of oral disease**
Tobacco prevention and cessation services reduce patient risks of developing tobacco-related oral diseases and conditions and improves prognosis for certain dental therapies.

● **D1321** **counseling for the control and prevention of adverse oral, behavioral, and systemic health effects associated with high-risk substance use**
Counseling services may include patient education about adverse oral, behavioral, and systemic effects associated with high-risk substance use and administration routes. This includes ingesting, injecting, inhaling and vaping. Substances used in a high-risk manner may include but are not limited to alcohol, opioids, nicotine, cannabis, methamphetamine and other pharmaceuticals or chemicals.

    ● new procedure code   ▲ revision to a nomenclature or descriptor # Editorial

D1330   **oral hygiene instructions**
This may include instructions for home care. Examples include tooth brushing technique, flossing, and use of special oral hygiene aids.

D1351   **sealant – per tooth**
Mechanically and/or chemically prepared enamel surface sealed to prevent decay.

D1353   **sealant repair – per tooth**

D1352   **preventive resin restoration in a moderate to high caries risk patient – permanent tooth**
Conservative restoration of an active cavitated lesion in a pit or fissure that does not extend into dentin; includes placement of a sealant in any radiating non-carious fissures or pits.

D1354   **interim caries arresting medicament application – per tooth**
Conservative treatment of an active, non-symptomatic carious lesion by topical application of a caries arresting or inhibiting medicament and without mechanical removal of sound tooth structure.

● **D1355**   **caries preventive medicament application – per tooth**
For primary prevention or remineralization. Medicaments applied do not include topical fluorides.

Space Maintenance (Passive Appliances)

Passive appliances are designed to prevent tooth movement.

D1510   **space maintainer – fixed, unilateral – per quadrant**
Excludes a distal shoe space maintainer.

D1516   **space maintainer – fixed – bilateral, maxillary**

D1517   **space maintainer – fixed – bilateral, mandibular**

D1520   **space maintainer – removable, unilateral – per quadrant**

D1526   **space maintainer – removable – bilateral, maxillary**

D1527   **space maintainer – removable – bilateral, mandibular**

D1551   **re-cement or re-bond bilateral space maintainer – maxillary**

D1552   **re-cement or re-bond bilateral space maintainer – mandibular**

D1553 re-cement or re-bond unilateral space maintainer – per quadrant

D1556 removal of fixed unilateral space maintainer – per quadrant

▲ **D1557** removal of fixed bilateral space maintainer – maxillary

▲ **D1558** removal of fixed bilateral space maintainer – mandibular

Space Maintainers

D1575 distal shoe space maintainer – fixed, unilateral – per quadrant
Fabrication and delivery of fixed appliance extending subgingivally and distally to guide the eruption of the first permanent molar. Does not include ongoing follow-up or adjustments, or replacement appliances, once the tooth has erupted.

D1999 unspecified preventive procedure, by report
Used for a procedure that is not adequately described by a code. Describe the procedure.

D2000–D2999 III. Restorative

Local anesthesia is usually considered to be part of Restorative procedures.

Explanation of Restorations

Location	Number of Surfaces	Characteristics
Anterior	1	Placed on one of the following five surface classifications – Mesial, Distal, Incisal, Lingual, or Facial (or Labial).
	2	Placed, without interruption, on two of the five surface classifications – e.g., Mesial-Lingual.
	3	Placed, without interruption, on three of the five surface classifications – e.g., Lingual-Mesial-Facial (or Labial).
	4 or more	Placed, without interruption, on four or more of the five surface classifications – e.g., Mesial-Incisal-Lingual-Facial (or Labial).
Posterior	1	Placed on one of the following five surface classifications – Mesial, Distal, Occlusal, Lingual, or Buccal.
	2	Placed, without interruption, on two of the five surface classifications – e.g., Mesial-Occlusal.
	3	Placed, without interruption, on three of the five surface classifications – e.g., Lingual-Occlusal-Distal.
	4 or more	Placed, without interruption, on four or more of the five surface classifications – e.g., Mesial-Occlusal-Lingual-Distal.

Note: Tooth surfaces are reported on the HIPAA standard electronic dental transaction and the ADA Dental Claim Form using the letters in the following table.

Surface	Code
Buccal	B
Distal	D
Facial (or Labial)	F
Incisal	I
Lingual	L
Mesial	M
Occlusal	O

Amalgam Restorations (Including Polishing)

Tooth preparation, all adhesives (including amalgam bonding agents), liners and bases are included as part of the restoration. If pins are used, they should be reported separately (see D2951).

D2140 **amalgam – one surface, primary or permanent**

D2150 **amalgam – two surfaces, primary or permanent**

D2160 **amalgam – three surfaces, primary or permanent**

D2161 **amalgam – four or more surfaces, primary or permanent**

Resin-Based Composite Restorations – Direct

Resin-based composite refers to a broad category of materials including but not limited to composites. May include bonded composite, light-cured composite, etc. Tooth preparation, acid etching, adhesives (including resin bonding agents), liners and bases and curing are included as part of the restoration. Glass ionomers, when used as restorations, should be reported with these codes. If pins are used, they should be reported separately (see D2951).

D2330 **resin-based composite – one surface, anterior**

D2331 **resin-based composite – two surfaces, anterior**

D2332 **resin-based composite – three surfaces, anterior**

D2335 **resin-based composite – four or more surfaces or involving incisal angle (anterior)**
Incisal angle to be defined as one of the angles formed by the junction of the incisal and the mesial or distal surface of an anterior tooth.

D2390 **resin-based composite crown, anterior**
Full resin-based composite coverage of tooth.

D2391 **resin-based composite – one surface, posterior**
Used to restore a carious lesion into the dentin or a deeply eroded area into the dentin. Not a preventive procedure.

D2392 **resin-based composite – two surfaces, posterior**

D2393 **resin-based composite – three surfaces, posterior**

D2394 **resin-based composite – four or more surfaces, posterior**

Gold Foil Restorations

D2410	**gold foil – one surface**
D2420	**gold foil – two surfaces**
D2430	**gold foil – three surfaces**

Inlay/Onlay Restorations

Inlay: An intra-coronal dental restoration, made outside the oral cavity to conform to the prepared cavity, which does not restore any cusp tips.

Onlay: A dental restoration made outside the oral cavity that covers one or more cusp tips and adjoining occlusal surfaces, but not the entire external surface.

D2510	**inlay – metallic – one surface**
D2520	**inlay – metallic – two surfaces**
D2530	**inlay – metallic – three or more surfaces**
D2542	**onlay – metallic – two surfaces**
D2543	**onlay – metallic – three surfaces**
D2544	**onlay – metallic – four or more surfaces**

Porcelain/ceramic inlays/onlays include all indirect ceramic and porcelain type inlays/onlays.

D2610	**inlay – porcelain/ceramic – one surface**
D2620	**inlay – porcelain/ceramic – two surfaces**
D2630	**inlay – porcelain/ceramic – three or more surfaces**
D2642	**onlay – porcelain/ceramic – two surfaces**
D2643	**onlay – porcelain/ceramic – three surfaces**
D2644	**onlay – porcelain/ceramic – four or more surfaces**

Resin-based composite inlays/onlays must utilize indirect technique.

D2650	**inlay – resin-based composite – one surface**
D2651	**inlay – resin-based composite – two surfaces**
D2652	**inlay – resin-based composite – three or more surfaces**

D2662	onlay – resin-based composite – two surfaces
D2663	onlay – resin-based composite – three surfaces
D2664	onlay – resin-based composite – four or more surfaces

Crowns – Single Restorations Only

D2710	crown – resin-based composite (indirect)
D2712	crown – ¾ resin-based composite (indirect) This procedure does not include facial veneers.
D2720	crown – resin with high noble metal
D2721	crown – resin with predominantly base metal
D2722	crown – resin with noble metal
D2740	crown – porcelain/ceramic
D2750	crown – porcelain fused to high noble metal
D2751	crown – porcelain fused to predominantly base metal
D2752	crown – porcelain fused to noble metal
D2753	crown – porcelain fused to titanium and titanium alloys
D2780	crown – ¾ cast high noble metal
D2781	crown – ¾ cast predominantly base metal
D2782	crown – ¾ cast noble metal
D2783	crown – ¾ porcelain/ceramic This procedure does not include facial veneers.
D2790	crown – full cast high noble metal
D2791	crown – full cast predominantly base metal
D2792	crown – full cast noble metal
D2794	crown – titanium and titanium alloys
D2799	provisional crown– further treatment or completion of diagnosis necessary prior to final impression Not to be used as a temporary crown for a routine prosthetic restoration.

 | ● new procedure code ▲ revision to a nomenclature or descriptor # Editorial

Other Restorative Services

D2990 **resin infiltration of incipient smooth surface lesions**
Placement of an infiltrating resin restoration for strengthening, stabilizing and/or limiting the progression of the lesion.

D2910 **re-cement or re-bond inlay, onlay, veneer or partial coverage restoration**

D2915 **re-cement or re-bond indirectly fabricated or prefabricated post and core**

D2920 **re-cement or re-bond crown**

D2921 **reattachment of tooth fragment, incisal edge or cusp**

D2929 **prefabricated porcelain/ceramic crown – primary tooth**

• **D2928** **prefabricated porcelain/ceramic crown – permanent tooth**

D2930 **prefabricated stainless steel crown – primary tooth**

D2931 **prefabricated stainless steel crown – permanent tooth**

D2932 **prefabricated resin crown**

D2933 **prefabricated stainless steel crown with resin window**
Open-face stainless steel crown with aesthetic resin facing or veneer.

D2934 **prefabricated esthetic coated stainless steel crown – primary tooth**
Stainless steel primary crown with exterior esthetic coating.

D2940 **protective restoration**
Direct placement of a restorative material to protect tooth and/ or tissue form. This procedure may be used to relieve pain, promote healing, or prevent further deterioration. Not to be used for endodontic access closure, or as a base or liner under restoration.

D2941 **interim therapeutic restoration – primary dentition**
Placement of an adhesive restorative material following caries debridement by hand or other method for the management of early childhood caries. Not considered a definitive restoration.

D2949 **restorative foundation for an indirect restoration**
Placement of restorative material to yield a more ideal form, including elimination of undercuts.

D2950 **core buildup, including any pins when required**
Refers to building up of coronal structure when there is insufficient retention for a separate extracoronal restorative procedure. A core buildup is not a filler to eliminate any undercut, box form, or concave irregularity in a preparation.

D2951	pin retention – per tooth, in addition to restoration
D2952	post and core in addition to crown, indirectly fabricated
	Post and core are custom fabricated as a single unit.
D2953	each additional indirectly fabricated post – same tooth
	To be used with D2952.
D2954	prefabricated post and core in addition to crown
	Core is built around a prefabricated post. This procedure includes the core material.
D2957	each additional prefabricated post – same tooth
	To be used with D2954.
D2955	post removal
# D2960	labial veneer (resin laminate) – direct
	Refers to labial/facial direct resin bonded veneers.
# D2961	labial veneer (resin laminate) – indirect
	Refers to labial/facial indirect resin bonded veneers.
# D2962	labial veneer (porcelain laminate) – indirect
	Refers also to facial veneers that extend interproximally and/or cover the incisal edge. Porcelain/ceramic veneers presently include all ceramic and porcelain veneers.
D2971	additional procedures to construct new crown under existing partial denture framework
	To be reported in addition to a crown code.
D2975	coping
	A thin covering of the coronal portion of a tooth, usually devoid of anatomic contour, that can be used as a definitive restoration.
D2980	crown repair necessitated by restorative material failure
D2981	inlay repair necessitated by restorative material failure
D2982	onlay repair necessitated by restorative material failure
D2983	veneer repair necessitated by restorative material failure
D2999	unspecified restorative procedure, by report
	Use for a procedure that is not adequately described by a code. Describe the procedure.

D3000–D3999 IV. Endodontics

Local anesthesia is usually considered to be part of Endodontic procedures.

Pulp Capping

D3110 pulp cap – direct (excluding final restoration)
Procedure in which the exposed pulp is covered with a dressing or cement that protects the pulp and promotes healing and repair.

D3120 pulp cap – indirect (excluding final restoration)
Procedure in which the nearly exposed pulp is covered with a protective dressing to protect the pulp from additional injury and to promote healing and repair via formation of secondary dentin. This code is not to be used for bases and liners when all caries has been removed.

Pulpotomy

D3220 therapeutic pulpotomy (excluding final restoration) – removal of pulp coronal to the dentinocemental junction and application of medicament
Pulpotomy is the surgical removal of a portion of the pulp with the aim of maintaining the vitality of the remaining portion by means of an adequate dressing.

– To be performed on primary or permanent teeth.

– This is not to be construed as the first stage of root canal therapy.

– Not to be used for apexogenesis.

D3221 pulpal debridement, primary and permanent teeth
Pulpal debridement for the relief of acute pain prior to conventional root canal therapy. This procedure is not to be used when endodontic treatment is completed on the same day.

D3222 partial pulpotomy for apexogenesis – permanent tooth with incomplete root development
Removal of a portion of the pulp and application of a medicament with the aim of maintaining the vitality of the remaining portion to encourage continued physiological development and formation of the root. This procedure is not to be construed as the first stage of root canal therapy.

Endodontic Therapy on Primary Teeth

Endodontic therapy on primary teeth with succedaneous teeth and placement of resorbable filling. This includes pulpectomy, cleaning, and filling of canals with resorbable material.

D3230 **pulpal therapy (resorbable filling) – anterior, primary tooth (excluding final restoration)**
Primary incisors and cuspids.

D3240 **pulpal therapy (resorbable filling) – posterior, primary tooth (excluding final restoration)**
Primary first and second molars.

Endodontic Therapy (Including Treatment Plan, Clinical Procedures and Follow-Up Care)

Includes primary teeth without succedaneous teeth and permanent teeth. Complete root canal therapy; pulpectomy is part of root canal therapy.

Includes all appointments necessary to complete treatment; also includes intra-operative radiographs. Does not include diagnostic evaluation and necessary radiographs/diagnostic images.

D3310 **endodontic therapy, anterior tooth (excluding final restoration)**

D3320 **endodontic therapy, premolar tooth (excluding final restoration)**

D3330 **endodontic therapy, molar tooth (excluding final restoration)**

D3331 **treatment of root canal obstruction; non-surgical access**
In lieu of surgery, the formation of a pathway to achieve an apical seal without surgical intervention because of a non-negotiable root canal blocked by foreign bodies, including but not limited to separated instruments, broken posts or calcification of 50% or more of the length of the tooth root.

D3332 **incomplete endodontic therapy; inoperable, unrestorable or fractured tooth**
Considerable time is necessary to determine diagnosis and/or provide initial treatment before the fracture makes the tooth unretainable.

D3333 **internal root repair of perforation defects**
Non-surgical seal of perforation caused by resorption and/or decay but not iatrogenic by provider filing claim.

Endodontic Retreatment

D3346   **retreatment of previous root canal therapy – anterior**

D3347   **retreatment of previous root canal therapy – premolar**

D3348   **retreatment of previous root canal therapy – molar**

Apexification/Recalcification

D3351   **apexification/recalcification – initial visit (apical closure/calcific repair of perforations, root resorption, etc.)**
Includes opening tooth, preparation of canal spaces, first placement of medication and necessary radiographs. (This procedure may include first phase of complete root canal therapy.)

D3352   **apexification/recalcification – interim medication replacement**
For visits in which the intra-canal medication is replaced with new medication. Includes any necessary radiographs.

D3353   **apexification/recalcification – final visit (includes completed root canal therapy – apical closure/calcific repair of perforations, root resorption, etc.)**
Includes removal of intra-canal medication and procedures necessary to place final root canal filling material including necessary radiographs. (This procedure includes last phase of complete root canal therapy.)

Pulpal Regeneration

D3355   **pulpal regeneration – initial visit**
Includes opening tooth, preparation of canal spaces, placement of medication.

D3356   **pulpal regeneration – interim medication replacement**

D3357   **pulpal regeneration – completion of treatment**
Does not include final restoration.

Apicoectomy/Periradicular Services

Periradicular surgery is a term used to describe surgery to the root surface (e.g., apicoectomy), repair of a root perforation or resorptive defect, exploratory curettage to look for root fractures, removal of extruded filling materials or instruments, removal of broken root fragments, sealing of accessory canals, etc. This does not include retrograde filling material placement.

D3410 **apicoectomy – anterior**
For surgery on root of anterior tooth. Does not include placement of retrograde filling material.

D3421 **apicoectomy – premolar (first root)**
For surgery on one root of a premolar. Does not include placement of retrograde filling material. If more than one root is treated, see D3426.

D3425 **apicoectomy – molar (first root)**
For surgery on one root of a molar tooth. Does not include placement of retrograde filling material. If more than one root is treated, see D3426.

D3426 **apicoectomy (each additional root)**
Typically used for premolar and molar surgeries when more than one root is treated during the same procedure. This does not include retrograde filling material placement.

● **D3471** **surgical repair of root resorption – anterior**
For surgery on root of anterior tooth. Does not include placement of restoration.

● **D3472** **surgical repair of root resorption – premolar**
For surgery on root of premolar tooth. Does not include placement of restoration.

● **D3473** **surgical repair of root resorption – molar**
For surgery on root of molar tooth. Does not include placement of restoration.

● **D3501** **surgical exposure of root surface without apicoectomy or repair of root resorption – anterior**
Exposure of root surface followed by observation and surgical closure of the exposed area. Not to be used for or in conjunction with apicoectomy or repair of root resorption.

- **D3502** **surgical exposure of root surface without apicoectomy or repair of root resorption – premolar**
  Exposure of root surface followed by observation and surgical closure of the exposed area. Not to be used for or in conjunction with apicoectomy or repair of root resorption.

- **D3503** **surgical exposure of root surface without apicoectomy or repair of root resorption – molar**
  Exposure of root surface followed by observation and surgical closure of the exposed area. Not to be used for or in conjunction with apicoectomy or repair of root resorption.

D3428 **bone graft in conjunction with periradicular surgery – per tooth, single site**
Includes non-autogenous graft material.

D3429 **bone graft in conjunction with periradicular surgery – each additional contiguous tooth in the same surgical site**
Includes non-autogenous graft material.

D3430 **retrograde filling – per root**
For placement of retrograde filling material during periradicular surgery procedures. If more than one filling is placed in one root report as D3999 and describe.

D3431 **biologic materials to aid in soft and osseous tissue regeneration in conjunction with periradicular surgery**

D3432 **guided tissue regeneration, resorbable barrier, per site, in conjunction with periradicular surgery**

D3450 **root amputation – per root**
Root resection of a multi-rooted tooth while leaving the crown. If the crown is sectioned, see D3920.

D3460 **endodontic endosseous implant**
Placement of implant material, which extends from a pulpal space into the bone beyond the end of the root.

D3470 **intentional re-implantation (including necessary splinting)**
For the intentional removal, inspection and treatment of the root and replacement of a tooth into its own socket. This does not include necessary retrograde filling material placement.

Other Endodontic Procedures

D3910 **surgical procedure for isolation of tooth with rubber dam**

D3920 **hemisection (including any root removal), not including root canal therapy**
Includes separation of a multi-rooted tooth into separate sections containing the root and the overlying portion of the crown. It may also include the removal of one or more of those sections.

D3950 **canal preparation and fitting of preformed dowel or post**
Should not be reported in conjunction with D2952, D2953, D2954 or D2957 by the same practitioner.

D3999 **unspecified endodontic procedure, by report**
Used for a procedure that is not adequately described by a code. Describe the procedure.

D4000–D4999 V. Periodontics

Local anesthesia is usually considered to be part of Periodontal procedures.

Surgical Services (Including Usual Postoperative Care)

Site: A term used to describe a single area, position, or locus. The word "site" is frequently used to indicate an area of soft tissue recession on a single tooth or an osseous defect adjacent to a single tooth; also used to indicate soft tissue defects and/or osseous defects in edentulous tooth positions.

- If two contiguous teeth have areas of soft tissue recession, each tooth is a single site.
- If two contiguous teeth have adjacent but separate osseous defects, each defect is a single site.
- If two contiguous teeth have a communicating interproximal osseous defect, it should be considered a single site.
- All non-communicating osseous defects are single sites.
- All edentulous non-contiguous tooth positions are single sites.
- Up to two contiguous edentulous tooth positions may be considered a single site.

Tooth Bounded Space: A space created by one or more missing teeth that has a tooth on each side.

D4210 **gingivectomy or gingivoplasty – four or more contiguous teeth or tooth bounded spaces per quadrant**
It is performed to eliminate suprabony pockets or to restore normal architecture when gingival enlargements or asymmetrical or unaesthetic topography is evident with normal bony configuration.

D4211 **gingivectomy or gingivoplasty – one to three contiguous teeth or tooth bounded spaces per quadrant**
It is performed to eliminate suprabony pockets or to restore normal architecture when gingival enlargements or asymmetrical or unaesthetic topography is evident with normal bony configuration.

D4212 **gingivectomy or gingivoplasty to allow access for restorative procedure, per tooth**

D4230   **anatomical crown exposure – four or more contiguous teeth or bounded tooth spaces per quadrant**
This procedure is utilized in an otherwise periodontally healthy area to remove enlarged gingival tissue and supporting bone (ostectomy) to provide an anatomically correct gingival relationship.

D4231   **anatomical crown exposure – one to three teeth or bounded tooth spaces per quadrant**
This procedure is utilized in an otherwise periodontally healthy area to remove enlarged gingival tissue and supporting bone (ostectomy) to provide an anatomically correct gingival relationship.

D4240   **gingival flap procedure, including root planing – four or more contiguous teeth or tooth bounded spaces per quadrant**
A soft tissue flap is reflected or resected to allow debridement of the root surface and the removal of granulation tissue. Osseous recontouring is not accomplished in conjunction with this procedure. May include open flap curettage, reverse bevel flap surgery, modified Kirkland flap procedure, and modified Widman surgery. This procedure is performed in the presence of moderate to deep probing depths, loss of attachment, need to maintain esthetics, need for increased access to the root surface and alveolar bone, or to determine the presence of a cracked tooth, fractured root, or external root resorption. Other procedures may be required concurrent to D4240 and should be reported separately using their own unique codes.

D4241   **gingival flap procedure, including root planing – one to three contiguous teeth or tooth bounded spaces per quadrant**
A soft tissue flap is reflected or resected to allow debridement of the root surface and the removal of granulation tissue. Osseous recontouring is not accomplished in conjunction with this procedure. May include open flap curettage, reverse bevel flap surgery, modified Kirkland flap procedure, and modified Widman surgery. This procedure is performed in the presence of moderate to deep probing depths, loss of attachment, need to maintain esthetics, need for increased access to the root surface and alveolar bone, or to determine the presence of a cracked tooth, fractured root, or external root resorption. Other procedures may be required concurrent to D4241 and should be reported separately using their own unique codes.

D4245   **apically positioned flap**
Procedure is used to preserve keratinized gingiva in conjunction with osseous resection and second stage implant procedure. Procedure may also be used to preserve keratinized/attached gingiva during surgical exposure of labially impacted teeth, and may be used during treatment of peri-implantitis.

D4249   **clinical crown lengthening – hard tissue**
This procedure is employed to allow a restorative procedure on a tooth with little or no tooth structure exposed to the oral cavity. Crown lengthening requires reflection of a full thickness flap and removal of bone, altering the crown to root ratio. It is performed in a healthy periodontal environment, as opposed to osseous surgery, which is performed in the presence of periodontal disease.

D4260   **osseous surgery (including elevation of a full thickness flap and closure) – four or more contiguous teeth or tooth bounded spaces per quadrant**
This procedure modifies the bony support of the teeth by reshaping the alveolar process to achieve a more physiologic form during the surgical procedure. This must include the removal of supporting bone (ostectomy) and/or non-supporting bone (osteoplasty). Other procedures may be required concurrent to D4260 and should be reported using their own unique codes.

D4261   **osseous surgery (including elevation of a full thickness flap and closure) – one to three contiguous teeth or tooth bounded spaces per quadrant**
This procedure modifies the bony support of the teeth by reshaping the alveolar process to achieve a more physiologic form during the surgical procedure. This must include the removal of supporting bone (ostectomy) and/or non-supporting bone (osteoplasty). Other procedures may be required concurrent to D4261 and should be reported using their own unique codes.

D4263   **bone replacement graft – retained natural tooth – first site in quadrant**
This procedure involves the use of grafts to stimulate periodontal regeneration when the disease process has led to a deformity of the bone. This procedure does not include flap entry and closure, wound debridement, osseous contouring, or the placement of biologic materials to aid in osseous tissue regeneration or barrier membranes. Other separate procedures delivered concurrently are documented with their own codes. Not to be reported for an edentulous space or an extraction site.

D4264 **bone replacement graft – retained natural tooth – each additional site in quadrant**
This procedure involves the use of grafts to stimulate periodontal regeneration when the disease process has led to a deformity of the bone. This procedure does not include flap entry and closure, wound debridement, osseous contouring, or the placement of biologic materials to aid in osseous tissue regeneration or barrier membranes. This procedure is performed concurrently with one or more bone replacement grafts to document the number of sites involved. Not to be reported for an edentulous space or an extraction site.

D4265 **biologic materials to aid in soft and osseous tissue regeneration**
Biologic materials may be used alone or with other regenerative substrates such as bone and barrier membranes, depending upon their formulation and the presentation of the periodontal defect. This procedure does not include surgical entry and closure, wound debridement, osseous contouring, or the placement of graft materials and/or barrier membranes. Other separate procedures may be required concurrent to D4265 and should be reported using their own unique codes.

D4266 **guided tissue regeneration – resorbable barrier, per site**
This procedure does not include flap entry and closure, or, when indicated, wound debridement, osseous contouring, bone replacement grafts, and placement of biologic materials to aid in osseous regeneration. This procedure can be used for periodontal and peri-implant defects.

D4267 **guided tissue regeneration – non-resorbable barrier, per site (includes membrane removal)**
This procedure does not include flap entry and closure, or, when indicated, wound debridement, osseous contouring, bone replacement grafts, and placement of biologic materials to aid in osseous regeneration. This procedure can be used for periodontal and peri-implant defects.

D4268 **surgical revision procedure, per tooth**
This procedure is to refine the results of a previously provided surgical procedure. This may require a surgical procedure to modify the irregular contours of hard or soft tissue. A mucoperiosteal flap may be elevated to allow access to reshape alveolar bone. The flaps are replaced or repositioned and sutured.

D4270 **pedicle soft tissue graft procedure**
A pedicle flap of gingiva can be raised from an edentulous ridge, adjacent teeth, or from the existing gingiva on the tooth and moved laterally or coronally to replace alveolar mucosa as marginal tissue. The procedure can be used to cover an exposed root or to eliminate a gingival defect if the root is not too prominent in the arch.

D4273 **autogenous connective tissue graft procedure (including donor and recipient surgical sites) first tooth, implant or edentulous tooth position in graft**
There are two surgical sites. The recipient site utilizes a split thickness incision, retaining the overlapping flap of gingiva and/or mucosa. The connective tissue is dissected from a separate donor site leaving an epithelialized flap for closure.

D4283 **autogenous connective tissue graft procedure (including donor and recipient surgical sites) – each additional contiguous tooth, implant or edentulous tooth position in same graft site**
Used in conjunction with D4273.

D4275 **non-autogenous connective tissue graft (including recipient site and donor material) first tooth, implant, or edentulous tooth position in graft**
There is only a recipient surgical site utilizing split thickness incision, retaining the overlaying flap of gingiva and/or mucosa. A donor surgical site is not present.

D4285 **non-autogenous connective tissue graft procedure (including recipient surgical site and donor material) – each additional contiguous tooth, implant or edentulous tooth position in same graft site**
Used in conjunction with D4275.

D4274 **mesial/distal wedge procedure, single tooth (when not performed in conjunction with surgical procedures in the same anatomical area)**
This procedure is performed in an edentulous area adjacent to a tooth, allowing removal of a tissue wedge to gain access for debridement, permit close flap adaptation, and reduce pocket depths.

D4276 **combined connective tissue and double pedicle graft, per tooth**
Advanced gingival recession often cannot be corrected with a single procedure. Combined tissue grafting procedures are needed to achieve the desired outcome.

D4277 **free soft tissue graft procedure (including recipient and donor surgical sites) first tooth, implant, or edentulous tooth position in graft**

D4278 **free soft tissue graft procedure (including recipient and donor surgical sites) each additional contiguous tooth, implant, or edentulous tooth position in same graft site**
Used in conjunction with D4277.

Non-Surgical Periodontal Service

D4320 **provisional splinting – intracoronal**
This is an interim stabilization of mobile teeth. A variety of methods and appliances may be employed for this purpose. Identify the teeth involved.

D4321 **provisional splinting – extracoronal**
This is an interim stabilization of mobile teeth. A variety of methods and appliances may be employed for this purpose. Identify the teeth involved.

D4341 **periodontal scaling and root planing – four or more teeth per quadrant**
This procedure involves instrumentation of the crown and root surfaces of the teeth to remove plaque and calculus from these surfaces. It is indicated for patients with periodontal disease and is therapeutic, not prophylactic, in nature. Root planing is the definitive procedure designed for the removal of cementum and dentin that is rough, and/or permeated by calculus or contaminated with toxins or microorganisms. Some soft tissue removal occurs. This procedure may be used as a definitive treatment in some stages of periodontal disease and/or as a part of pre-surgical procedures in others.

D4342 **periodontal scaling and root planing – one to three teeth per quadrant**
This procedure involves instrumentation of the crown and root surfaces of the teeth to remove plaque and calculus from these surfaces. It is indicated for patients with periodontal disease and is therapeutic, not prophylactic, in nature. Root planing is the definitive procedure designed for the removal of cementum and dentin that is rough, and/or permeated by calculus or contaminated with toxins or microorganisms. Some soft tissue removal occurs. This procedure may be used as a definitive treatment in some stages of periodontal disease and/or as a part of pre-surgical procedures in others.

D4346 **scaling in presence of generalized moderate or severe gingival inflammation – full mouth, after oral evaluation**
The removal of plaque, calculus and stains from supra- and sub-gingival tooth surfaces when there is generalized moderate or severe gingival inflammation in the absence of periodontitis. It is indicated for patients who have swollen, inflamed gingiva, generalized suprabony pockets, and moderate to severe bleeding on probing. Should not be reported in conjunction with prophylaxis, scaling and root planing, or debridement procedures.

D4355 **full mouth debridement to enable a comprehensive oral evaluation and diagnosis on a subsequent visit**
Full mouth debridement involves the preliminary removal of plaque and calculus that interferes with the ability of the dentist to perform a comprehensive oral evaluation. Not to be completed on the same day as D0150, D0160, or D0180.

D4381 **localized delivery of antimicrobial agents via a controlled release vehicle into diseased crevicular tissue, per tooth**
FDA approved subgingival delivery devices containing antimicrobial medication(s) are inserted into periodontal pockets to suppress the pathogenic microbiota. These devices slowly release the pharmacological agents so they can remain at the intended site of action in a therapeutic concentration for a sufficient length of time.

Other Periodontal Services

D4910 **periodontal maintenance**
This procedure is instituted following periodontal therapy and continues at varying intervals, determined by the clinical evaluation of the dentist, for the life of the dentition or any implant replacements. It includes removal of the bacterial plaque and calculus from supragingival and subgingival regions, site specific scaling and root planing where indicated, and polishing the teeth. If new or recurring periodontal disease appears, additional diagnostic and treatment procedures must be considered.

D4920 **unscheduled dressing change (by someone other than treating dentist or their staff)**

D4921 **gingival irrigation – per quadrant**
Irrigation of gingival pockets with medicinal agent. Not to be used to report use of mouth rinses or non-invasive chemical debridement.

D4999 **unspecified periodontal procedure, by report**
Use for a procedure that is not adequately described by a code. Describe the procedure.

D5000–D5899 VI. Prosthodontics, removable

Local anesthesia is usually considered to be part of Removable Prosthodontic procedures.

Complete Dentures (Including Routine Post-Delivery Care)

D5110   **complete denture – maxillary**

D5120   **complete denture – mandibular**

D5130   **immediate denture – maxillary**
Includes limited follow-up care only; does not include future rebasing/relining procedure(s).

D5140   **immediate denture – mandibular**
Includes limited follow-up care only; does not include future rebasing/relining procedure(s).

Partial Dentures (Including Routine Post-Delivery Care)

D5211   **maxillary partial denture – resin base (including retentive/clasping materials, rests, and teeth)**

D5212   **mandibular partial denture – resin base (including retentive/clasping materials, rests, and teeth)**

D5213   **maxillary partial denture – cast metal framework with resin denture bases (including retentive/clasping materials, rests and teeth)**

D5214   **mandibular partial denture – cast metal framework with resin denture bases (including retentive/clasping materials, rests and teeth)**

D5221   **immediate maxillary partial denture – resin base (including retentive/clasping materials, rests and teeth)**
Includes limited follow-up care only; does not include future rebasing/relining procedure(s).

D5222   **immediate mandibular partial denture – resin base (including retentive/clasping materials, rests and teeth)**
Includes limited follow-up care only; does not include future rebasing/relining procedure(s).

D5223 **immediate maxillary partial denture – cast metal framework with resin denture bases (including retentive/clasping materials, rests and teeth)**
Includes limited follow-up care only; does not include future rebasing/relining procedure(s).

D5224 **immediate mandibular partial denture – cast metal framework with resin denture bases (including retentive/clasping materials, rests and teeth)**
Includes limited follow-up care only; does not include future rebasing/relining procedure(s).

\# **D5225** **maxillary partial denture – flexible base (including retentive/clasping materials, rests, and teeth)**

\# **D5226** **mandibular partial denture – flexible base (including retentive/clasping materials, rests, and teeth)**

\# **D5282** **removable unilateral partial denture – one piece cast metal (including retentive/clasping materials, rests, and teeth), maxillary**

\# **D5283** **removable unilateral partial denture – one piece cast metal (including retentive/clasping materials, rests, and teeth), mandibular**

\# **D5284** **removable unilateral partial denture – one piece flexible base (including retentive/clasping materials, rests, and teeth) – per quadrant**

\# **D5286** **removable unilateral partial denture – one piece resin (including retentive/clasping materials, rests, and teeth) – per quadrant**

Adjustments to Dentures

D5410 **adjust complete denture – maxillary**

D5411 **adjust complete denture – mandibular**

D5421 **adjust partial denture – maxillary**

D5422 **adjust partial denture – mandibular**

Repairs to Complete Dentures

D5511   repair broken complete denture base, mandibular

D5512   repair broken complete denture base, maxillary

D5520   replace missing or broken teeth – complete denture (each tooth)

Repairs to Partial Dentures

D5611   repair resin partial denture base, mandibular

D5612   repair resin partial denture base, maxillary

D5621   repair cast partial framework, mandibular

D5622   repair cast partial framework, maxillary

D5630   repair or replace broken retentive/clasping materials – per tooth

D5640   replace broken teeth – per tooth

D5650   add tooth to existing partial denture

D5660   add clasp to existing partial denture – per tooth

D5670   replace all teeth and acrylic on cast metal framework (maxillary)

D5671   replace all teeth and acrylic on cast metal framework (mandibular)

Denture Rebase Procedures
Rebase – process of refitting a denture by replacing the base material.

D5710   rebase complete maxillary denture

D5711   rebase complete mandibular denture

D5720   rebase maxillary partial denture

D5721   rebase mandibular partial denture

Denture Reline Procedures

Reline is the process of resurfacing the tissue side of a denture with new base material.

\# **D5730**   **reline complete maxillary denture (direct)**

\# **D5731**   **reline complete mandibular denture (direct)**

\# **D5740**   **reline maxillary partial denture (direct)**

\# **D5741**   **reline mandibular partial denture (direct)**

\# **D5750**   **reline complete maxillary denture (indirect)**

\# **D5751**   **reline complete mandibular denture (indirect)**

\# **D5760**   **reline maxillary partial denture (indirect)**

\# **D5761**   **reline mandibular partial denture (indirect)**

Interim Prosthesis

A provisional prosthesis designed for use over a limited period of time, after which it is to be replaced by a more definitive restoration.

D5810   **interim complete denture (maxillary)**

D5811   **interim complete denture (mandibular)**

\# **D5820**   **interim partial denture (including retentive/clasping materials, rests, and teeth), maxillary**

\# **D5821**   **interim partial denture (including retentive/clasping materials, rests, and teeth), mandibular**

Other Removable Prosthetic Services

D5850   **tissue conditioning, maxillary**
Treatment reline using materials designed to heal unhealthy ridges prior to more definitive final restoration.

D5851   **tissue conditioning, mandibular**
Treatment reline using materials designed to heal unhealthy ridges prior to more definitive final restoration.

D5862   **precision attachment, by report**
Each set of male and female components should be reported as one precision attachment. Describe the type of attachment used.

D5863	overdenture – complete maxillary
D5864	overdenture – partial maxillary
D5865	overdenture – complete mandibular
D5866	overdenture – partial mandibular
D5867	replacement of replaceable part of semi-precision or precision attachment (male or female component)
D5875	modification of removable prosthesis following implant surgery Attachment assemblies are reported using separate codes.
D5876	add metal substructure to acrylic full denture (per arch)
D5899	unspecified removable prosthodontic procedure, by report Use for a procedure that is not adequately described by a code. Describe the procedure.

D5900–D5999 VII. Maxillofacial Prosthetics

D5992   **adjust maxillofacial prosthetic appliance, by report**

D5993   **maintenance and cleaning of a maxillofacial prosthesis (extra- or intra-oral) other than required adjustments, by report**

D5914   **auricular prosthesis**
Synonymous terminology: artificial ear, ear prosthesis.

A removable prosthesis, which artificially restores part or all of the natural ear. Usually, replacement prostheses can be made from the original mold if tissue bed changes have not occurred. Creation of an auricular prosthesis requires fabrication of a mold, from which additional prostheses usually can be made, as needed later (auricular prosthesis, replacement).

D5927   **auricular prosthesis, replacement**
Synonymous terminology: replacement ear.

An artificial ear produced from a previously made mold. A replacement prosthesis does not require fabrication of a new mold. Generally, several prostheses can be made from the same mold assuming no changes occur in the tissue bed due to surgery or age related topographical variations.

D5987   **commissure splint**
Synonymous terminology: lip splint.

A device placed between the lips, which assists in achieving increased opening between the lips. Use of such devices enhances opening where surgical, chemical or electrical alterations of the lips has resulted in severe restriction or contractures.

D5924   **cranial prosthesis**
Synonymous terminology: Skull plate, cranioplasty prosthesis, cranial implant.

A biocompatible, permanently implanted replacement of a portion of the skull bones; an artificial replacement for a portion of the skull bone.

D5925   **facial augmentation implant prosthesis**
Synonymous terminology: facial implant.

An implantable biocompatible material generally onlayed upon an existing bony area beneath the skin tissue to fill in or collectively raise portions of the overlaying facial skin tissues to create acceptable contours.

Although some forms of pre-made surgical implants are commercially available, the facial augmentation is usually custom made for surgical implantation for each individual patient due to the irregular or extensive nature of the facial deficit.

D5912   facial moulage (complete)
Synonymous terminology: facial impression, face mask impression.

A complete facial moulage impression is a procedure used to record the soft tissue contours of the whole face. The impression is utilized to create a facial moulage and generally is not reusable.

D5911   facial moulage (sectional)
A sectional facial moulage impression is a procedure used to record the soft tissue contours of a portion of the face. Occasionally several separate sectional impressions are made, and then reassembled to provide a full facial contour cast. The impression is utilized to create a partial facial moulage and generally is not reusable.

D5919   facial prosthesis
Synonymous terminology: prosthetic dressing.

A removable prosthesis, which artificially replaces a portion of the face, lost due to surgery, trauma or congenital absence.

Flexion of natural tissues may preclude adaptation and movement of the prosthesis to match the adjacent skin. Salivary leakage, when communicating with the oral cavity, adversely affects retention.

D5929   facial prosthesis, replacement
A replacement facial prosthesis made from the original mold. A replacement prosthesis does not require fabrication of a new mold. Generally, several prostheses can be made from the same mold assuming no changes occur in the tissue bed due to further surgery or age related topographical variations.

D5951   feeding aid
Synonymous terminology: feeding prosthesis.

A prosthesis, which maintains the right and left maxillary segments of an infant cleft palate patient in their proper orientation until surgery is performed to repair the cleft. It closes the oral–nasal cavity defect, thus enhancing sucking and swallowing.

Used on an interim basis, this prosthesis achieves separation of the oral and nasal cavities in infants born with wide clefts necessitating delayed closure. It is eliminated if surgical closure can be effected or, alternatively, with eruption of the deciduous dentition a pediatric speech aid may be made to facilitate closure of the defect.

D5934 **mandibular resection prosthesis with guide flange**
Synonymous terminology: resection device, resection appliance.

A prosthesis which guides the remaining portion of the mandible, left after a partial resection, into a more normal relationship with the maxilla. This allows for some tooth-to-tooth or an improved tooth contact. It may also artificially replace missing teeth and thereby increase masticatory efficiency.

D5935 **mandibular resection prosthesis without guide flange**
A prosthesis which helps guide the partially resected mandible to a more normal relation with the maxilla allowing for increased tooth contact. It does not have a flange or ramp, however, to assist in directional closure. It may replace missing teeth and thereby increase masticatory efficiency.

Dentists who treat mandibulectomy patients may prefer to replace some, all or none of the teeth in the defect area. Frequently, the defect's margins preclude even partial replacement. Use of a guide (a mandibular resection prosthesis with a guide flange) may not be possible due to anatomical limitations or poor patient tolerance. Ramps, extended occlusal arrangements and irregular occlusal positioning relative to the denture foundation frequently preclude stability of the prostheses, and thus some prostheses are poorly tolerated under such adverse circumstances.

D5913 **nasal prosthesis**
Synonymous terminology: artificial nose.

A removable prosthesis attached to the skin, which artificially restores part or all of the nose. Fabrication of a nasal prosthesis requires creation of an original mold. Additional prostheses usually can be made from the same mold, and assuming no further tissue changes occur, the same mold can be utilized for extended periods of time.

When a new prosthesis is made from the existing mold, this procedure is termed a nasal prosthesis replacement.

D5926 **nasal prosthesis, replacement**
Synonymous terminology: replacement nose.

An artificial nose produced from a previously made mold. A replacement prosthesis does not require fabrication of a new mold. Generally, several prostheses can be made from the same mold assuming no changes occur in the tissue bed due to surgery or age related topographical variations.

D5922 **nasal septal prosthesis**
Synonymous terminology: Septal plug, septal button.

Removable prosthesis to occlude (obturate) a hole within the nasal septal wall. Adverse chemical degradation in this moist environment may require frequent replacement. Silicone prostheses are occasionally subject to fungal invasion.

D5932 **obturator prosthesis, definitive**
Synonymous terminology: obturator.

A prosthesis, which artificially replaces part or all of the maxilla and associated teeth, lost due to surgery, trauma or congenital defects.

A definitive obturator is made when it is deemed that further tissue changes or recurrence of tumor are unlikely and a more permanent prosthetic rehabilitation can be achieved; it is intended for long-term use.

D5936 **obturator prosthesis, interim**
Synonymous terminology: immediate postoperative obturator.

A prosthesis which is made following completion of the initial healing after a surgical resection of a portion or all of one or both the maxillae; frequently many or all teeth in the defect area are replaced by this prosthesis. This prosthesis replaces the surgical obturator, which is usually inserted at, or immediately following the resection.

Generally, an interim obturator is made to facilitate closure of the resultant defect after initial healing has been completed. Unlike the surgical obturator, which usually is made prior to surgery and frequently revised in the operating room during surgery, the interim obturator is made when the defect margins are clearly defined and further surgical revisions are not planned. It is a provisional prosthesis, which may replace some or all lost teeth, and other lost bone and soft tissue structures. Also, it frequently must be revised (termed an obturator prosthesis modification) during subsequent dental procedures (e.g., restorations, gingival surgery) as well as to compensate for further tissue shrinkage before a definitive obturator prosthesis is made.

D5933 **obturator prosthesis, modification**
Synonymous terminology: adjustment, denture adjustment, temporary or office reline.

Revision or alteration of an existing obturator (surgical, interim, or definitive); possible modifications include relief of the denture base due to tissue compression, augmentation of the seal or peripheral areas to effect adequate sealing or separation between the nasal and oral cavities.

  ● new procedure code ▲ revision to a nomenclature or descriptor # Editorial

D5931**obturator prosthesis, surgical**
Synonymous terminology: Obturator, surgical stayplate, immediate temporary obturator.

A temporary prosthesis inserted during or immediately following surgical or traumatic loss of a portion or all of one or both maxillary bones and contiguous alveolar structures (e.g., gingival tissue, teeth).

Frequent revisions of surgical obturators are necessary during the ensuing healing phase (approximately six months). Some dentists prefer to replace many or all teeth removed by the surgical procedure in the surgical obturator, while others do not replace any teeth. Further surgical revisions may require fabrication of another surgical obturator (e.g., an initially planned small defect may be revised and greatly enlarged after the final pathology report indicates margins are not free of tumor).

D5916**ocular prosthesis**
Synonymous terminology: artificial eye, glass eye.

A prosthesis, which artificially replaces an eye missing as a result of trauma, surgery or congenital absence. The prosthesis does not replace missing eyelids or adjacent skin, mucosa or muscle.

Ocular prostheses require semiannual or annual cleaning and polishing. Also, occasional revisions to re-adapt the prosthesis to the tissue bed may be necessary. Glass eyes are rarely made and cannot be re-adapted.

D5923**ocular prosthesis, interim**
Synonymous terminology: Eye shell, shell, ocular conformer, conformer.

A temporary replacement generally made of clear acrylic resin for an eye lost due to surgery or trauma. No attempt is made to re-establish esthetics. Fabrication of an interim ocular prosthesis generally implies subsequent fabrication of an aesthetic ocular prosthesis.

D5915**orbital prosthesis**
A prosthesis, which artificially restores the eye, eyelids, and adjacent hard and soft tissue, lost as a result of trauma or surgery.

Fabrication of an orbital prosthesis requires creation of an original mold. Additional prostheses usually can be made from the same mold, and assuming no further tissue changes occur, the same mold can be utilized for extended periods of time.

When a new prosthesis is made from the existing mold, this procedure is termed an orbital prosthesis replacement.

D5928   **orbital prosthesis, replacement**
A replacement for a previously made orbital prosthesis. A replacement prosthesis does not require fabrication of a new mold. Generally, several prostheses can be made from the same mold assuming no changes occur in the tissue bed due to surgery or age related topographical variations.

D5954   **palatal augmentation prosthesis**
Synonymous terminology: superimposed prosthesis, maxillary glossectomy prosthesis, maxillary speech prosthesis, palatal drop prosthesis.

A removable prosthesis which alters the hard and/or soft palate's topographical form adjacent to the tongue.

D5955   **palatal lift prosthesis, definitive**
A prosthesis which elevates the soft palate superiorly and aids in restoration of soft palate functions which may be lost due to an acquired, congenital or developmental defect.

A definitive palatal lift is usually made for patients whose experience with an interim palatal lift has been successful, especially if surgical alterations are deemed unwarranted.

D5958   **palatal lift prosthesis, interim**
Synonymous terminology: diagnostic palatal lift.

A prosthesis which elevates and assists in restoring soft palate function which may be lost due to clefting, surgery, trauma or unknown paralysis. It is intended for interim use to determine its usefulness in achieving palatalpharyngeal competency or enhance swallowing reflexes.

This prosthesis is intended for interim use as a diagnostic aid to assess the level of possible improvement in speech intelligibility. Some clinicians believe use of a palatal lift on an interim basis may stimulate an otherwise flaccid soft palate to increase functional activity, subsequently lessening its need.

D5959   **palatal lift prosthesis, modification**
Synonymous terminology: revision of lift, adjustment.

Alterations in the adaptation, contour, form or function of an existing palatal lift necessitated due to tissue impingement, lack of function, poor clasp adaptation or the like.

D5985   **radiation cone locator**
Synonymous terminology: docking device, cone locator.

A prosthesis utilized to direct and reduplicate the path of radiation to an oral tumor during a split course of irradiation.

D5984   radiation shield

Synonymous terminology: radiation stent, tongue protector, lead shield.

An intraoral prosthesis designed to shield adjacent tissues from radiation during orthovoltage treatment of malignant lesions of the head and neck region.

D5953   speech aid prosthesis, adult

Synonymous terminology: prosthetic speech appliance, speech aid, speech bulb.

A definitive prosthesis, which can improve speech in adult cleft palate patients either by obturating (sealing off) a palatal cleft or fistula, or occasionally by assisting an incompetent soft palate. Both mechanisms are necessary to achieve velopharyngeal competency.

Generally, this prosthesis is fabricated when no further growth is anticipated and the objective is to achieve long-term use. Hence, more precise materials and techniques are utilized. Occasionally such procedures are accomplished in conjunction with precision attachments in crown work undertaken on some or all maxillary teeth to achieve improved aesthetics.

D5960   speech aid prosthesis, modification

Synonymous terminology: adjustment, repair, revision.

Any revision of a pediatric or adult speech aid not necessitating its replacement.

Frequently, revisions of the obturating section of any speech aid are required to facilitate enhanced speech intelligibility. Such revisions or repairs do not require complete remaking of the prosthesis, thus extending its longevity.

D5952   speech aid prosthesis, pediatric

Synonymous terminology: nasopharyngeal obturator, speech appliance, obturator, cleft palate appliance, prosthetic speech aid, speech bulb.

A temporary or interim prosthesis used to close a defect in the hard and/or soft palate. It may replace tissue lost due to developmental or surgical alterations. It is necessary for the production of intelligible speech.

Normal lateral growth of the palatal bones necessitates occasional replacement of this prosthesis. Intermittent revisions of the obturator section can assist in maintenance of palatalpharyngeal closure (termed a speech aid prosthesis modification). Frequently, such prostheses are not fabricated before the deciduous dentition is fully erupted since clasp retention is often essential.

D5988 surgical splint
Synonymous terminology: Gunning splint, modified Gunning splint, labiolingual splint, fenestrated splint, Kingsley splint, cast metal splint.

Splints are designed to utilize existing teeth and/or alveolar processes as points of anchorage to assist in stabilization and immobilization of broken bones during healing. They are used to re-establish, as much as possible, normal occlusal relationships during the process of immobilization. Frequently, existing prostheses (e.g., a patient's complete dentures) can be modified to serve as surgical splints. Frequently, surgical splints have arch bars added to facilitate intermaxillary fixation. Rubber elastics may be used to assist in this process. Circummandibular eyelet hooks can be utilized for enhanced stabilization with wiring to adjacent bone.

D5982 surgical stent
Synonymous terminology: periodontal stent, skin graft stent, columellar stent.

Stents are utilized to apply pressure to soft tissues to facilitate healing and prevent cicatrization or collapse.

A surgical stent may be required in surgical and post-surgical revisions to achieve close approximation of tissues. Usually such materials as temporary or interim soft denture liners, gutta percha, or dental modeling impression compound may be used.

D5937 trismus appliance (not for TMD treatment)
Synonymous terminology: occlusal device for mandibular trismus, dynamic bite opener.

A prosthesis, which assists the patient in increasing their oral aperture width in order to eat as well as maintain oral hygiene.

Several versions and designs are possible, all intending to ease the severe lack of oral opening experienced by many patients immediately following extensive intraoral surgical procedures.

Carriers

D5986 fluoride gel carrier
Synonymous terminology: fluoride applicator.

A prosthesis, which covers the teeth in either dental arch and is used to apply topical fluoride in close proximity to tooth enamel and dentin for several minutes daily.

- **D5995** **periodontal medicament carrier with peripheral seal – laboratory processed – maxillary**
  A custom fabricated, laboratory processed carrier for the maxillary arch that covers the teeth and alveolar mucosa. Used as a vehicle to deliver prescribed medicaments for sustained contact with the gingiva, alveolar mucosa, and into the periodontal sulcus or pocket.

- **D5996** **periodontal medicament carrier with peripheral seal – laboratory processed – mandibular**
  A custom fabricated, laboratory processed carrier for the mandibular arch that covers the teeth and alveolar mucosa. Used as a vehicle to deliver prescribed medicaments for sustained contact with the gingiva, alveolar mucosa, and into the periodontal sulcus or pocket.

D5983 **radiation carrier**
Synonymous terminology: radiotherapy prosthesis, carrier prosthesis, radiation applicator, radium carrier, intracavity carrier, intracavity applicator.

A device used to administer radiation to confined areas by means of capsules, beads or needles of radiation emitting materials such as radium or cesium. Its function is to hold the radiation source securely in the same location during the entire period of treatment.

Radiation oncologists occasionally request these devices to achieve close approximation and controlled application of radiation to a tumor deemed amiable to eradication.

D5991 **vesiculobullous disease medicament carrier**
A custom fabricated carrier that covers the teeth and alveolar mucosa, or alveolar mucosa alone, and is used to deliver prescription medicaments for treatment of immunologically mediated vesiculobullous diseases.

D5999 **unspecified maxillofacial prosthesis, by report**
Used for a procedure that is not adequately described by a code. Describe the procedure.

D6000–D6199 VIII. Implant Services

Local anesthesia is usually considered to be part of Implant Services procedures.

Pre-Surgical Services

D6190 **radiographic/surgical implant index, by report**
An appliance, designed to relate osteotomy or fixture position to existing anatomic structures, to be utilized during radiographic exposure for treatment planning and/or during osteotomy creation for fixture installation.

Surgical Services

Report surgical implant procedure using codes in this section.

D6010 **surgical placement of implant body: endosteal implant**

▲ **D6011** **surgical access to an implant body (second stage implant surgery)**
This procedure, also known as second stage implant surgery, involves removal of tissue that covers the implant body so that a fixture of any type can be placed, or an existing fixture be replaced with another. Examples of fixtures include but are not limited to healing caps, abutments shaped to help contour the gingival margins or the final restorative prosthesis.

D6012 **surgical placement of interim implant body for transitional prosthesis: endosteal implant**
Includes removal during later therapy to accommodate the definitive restoration, which may include placement of other implants.

D6013 **surgical placement of mini implant**

D6040 **surgical placement: eposteal implant**
An eposteal (subperiosteal) framework of a biocompatible material designed and fabricated to fit on the surface of the bone of the mandible or maxilla with permucosal extensions which provide support and attachment of a prosthesis. This may be a complete arch or unilateral appliance. Eposteal implants rest upon the bone and under the periosteum.

 ● new procedure code ▲ revision to a nomenclature or descriptor # Editorial

D6050   **surgical placement: transosteal implant**
A transosteal (transosseous) biocompatible device with threaded posts penetrating both the superior and inferior cortical bone plates of the mandibular symphysis and exiting through the permucosa providing support and attachment for a dental prosthesis. Transosteal implants are placed completely through the bone and into the oral cavity from extraoral or intraoral.

D6100   **implant removal, by report**
This procedure involves the surgical removal of an implant.
Describe procedure.

D6101   **debridement of a peri-implant defect or defects surrounding a single implant, and surface cleaning of the exposed implant surfaces, including flap entry and closure**

D6102   **debridement and osseous contouring of a peri-implant defect or defects surrounding a single implant and includes surface cleaning of the exposed implant surfaces, including flap entry and closure**

D6103   **bone graft for repair of peri-implant defect – does not include flap entry and closure**
Placement of a barrier membrane or biologic materials to aid in osseous regeneration, are reported separately.

D6104   **bone graft at time of implant placement**
Placement of a barrier membrane, or biologic materials to aid in osseous regeneration are reported separately.

Implant Supported Prosthetics

Supporting Structures

D6055   **connecting bar – implant supported or abutment supported**
Utilized to stabilize and anchor a prosthesis.

D6056   **prefabricated abutment – includes modification and placement**
Modification of a prefabricated abutment may be necessary.

D6057   **custom fabricated abutment – includes placement**
Created by a laboratory process, specific for an individual application.

D6051   **interim abutment**
Includes placement and removal. A healing cap is not an interim abutment.

- **D6191** **semi-precision abutment – placement**
  This procedure is the initial placement, or replacement, of a semi-precision abutment on the implant body.

- **D6192** **semi-precision attachment – placement**
  This procedure involves the luting of the initial, or replacement, semi-precision attachment to the removable prosthesis.

Implant/Abutment Supported Removable Dentures

D6110 **implant/abutment supported removable denture for edentulous arch – maxillary**

D6111 **implant/abutment supported removable denture for edentulous arch – mandibular**

D6112 **implant/abutment supported removable denture for partially edentulous arch – maxillary**

D6113 **implant/abutment supported removable denture for partially edentulous arch – mandibular**

Implant/Abutment Supported Fixed Dentures (Hybrid Prosthesis)

D6114 **implant/abutment supported fixed denture for edentulous arch – maxillary**

D6115 **implant/abutment supported fixed denture for edentulous arch – mandibular**

D6116 **implant/abutment supported fixed denture for partially edentulous arch – maxillary**

D6117 **implant/abutment supported fixed denture for partially edentulous arch – mandibular**

D6118 **implant/abutment supported interim fixed denture for edentulous arch – mandibular**
  Used when a period of healing is necessary prior to fabrication and placement of a permanent prosthetic.

D6119 **implant/abutment supported interim fixed denture for edentulous arch – maxillary**
  Used when a period of healing is necessary prior to fabrication and placement of a permanent prosthetic.

Single Crowns, Abutment Supported

D6058   abutment supported porcelain/ceramic crown
A single crown restoration that is retained, supported and stabilized by an abutment on an implant.

D6059   abutment supported porcelain fused to metal crown (high noble metal)
A single metal-ceramic crown restoration that is retained, supported and stabilized by an abutment on an implant.

D6060   abutment supported porcelain fused to metal crown (predominantly base metal)
A single metal-ceramic crown restoration that is retained, supported and stabilized by an abutment on an implant.

D6061   abutment supported porcelain fused to metal crown (noble metal)
A single metal-ceramic crown restoration that is retained, supported and stabilized by an abutment on an implant.

D6097   abutment supported crown – porcelain fused to titanium or titanium alloys
A single metal-ceramic crown restoration that is retained, supported, and stabilized by an abutment on an implant.

D6062   abutment supported cast metal crown (high noble metal)
A single cast metal crown restoration that is retained, supported and stabilized by an abutment on an implant.

D6063   abutment supported cast metal crown (predominantly base metal)
A single cast metal crown restoration that is retained, supported and stabilized by an abutment on an implant.

D6064   abutment supported cast metal crown (noble metal)
A single cast metal crown restoration that is retained, supported and stabilized by an abutment on an implant.

D6094   abutment supported crown titanium and titanium alloys
A single crown restoration that is retained, supported and stabilized by an abutment on an implant.

D6065   **implant supported porcelain/ceramic crown**
A single crown restoration that is retained, supported and stabilized by an implant.

D6066   **implant supported crown – porcelain fused to high noble alloys**
A single metal-ceramic crown restoration that is retained, supported and stabilized by an implant.

D6082   **implant supported crown – porcelain fused to predominantly base alloys**
A single metal-ceramic crown restoration that is retained, supported and stabilized by an implant.

D6083   **implant supported crown – porcelain fused to noble alloys**
A single metal-ceramic crown restoration that is retained, supported and stabilized by an implant.

D6084   **implant supported crown – porcelain fused to titanium or titanium alloys**
A single metal-ceramic crown restoration that is retained, supported and stabilized by an implant.

D6067   **implant supported crown - high noble alloys**
A single metal crown restoration that is retained, supported and stabilized by an implant.

D6086   **implant supported crown – predominantly base alloys**
A single metal crown restoration that is retained, supported and stabilized by an implant.

D6087   **implant supported crown – noble alloys**
A single metal crown restoration that is retained, supported and stabilized by an implant.

D6088   **implant supported crown – titanium and titanium alloys**
A single metal crown restoration that is retained, supported and stabilized by an implant.

● new procedure code   ▲ revision to a nomenclature or descriptor   # Editorial

Fixed Partial Denture (FPD) Retainer, Abutment Supported

D6068 **abutment supported retainer for porcelain/ceramic FPD**
A ceramic retainer for a fixed partial denture that gains retention, support and stability from an abutment on an implant.

D6069 **abutment supported retainer for porcelain fused to metal FPD (high noble metal)**
A metal-ceramic retainer for a fixed partial denture that gains retention, support and stability from an abutment on an implant.

D6070 **abutment supported retainer for porcelain fused to metal FPD (predominantly base metal)**
A metal-ceramic retainer for a fixed partial denture that gains retention, support and stability from an abutment on an implant.

D6071 **abutment supported retainer for porcelain fused to metal FPD (noble metal)**
A metal-ceramic retainer for a fixed partial denture that gains retention, support and stability from an abutment on an implant.

D6195 **abutment supported retainer – porcelain fused to titanium and titanium alloys**
A metal-ceramic retainer for a fixed partial denture that gains retention, support, and stability from an abutment on an implant.

D6072 **abutment supported retainer for cast metal FPD (high noble metal)**
A cast metal retainer for a fixed partial denture that gains retention, support and stability from an abutment on an implant.

D6073 **abutment supported retainer for cast metal FPD (predominantly base metal)**
A cast metal retainer for a fixed partial denture that gains retention, support and stability from an abutment on an implant.

D6074 **abutment supported retainer for cast metal FPD (noble metal)**
A cast metal retainer for a fixed partial denture that gains retention, support and stability from an abutment on an implant.

D6194 **abutment supported retainer crown for FPD – titanium and titanium alloys**
A retainer for a fixed partial denture that gains retention, support and stability from an abutment on an implant.

D6075 **implant supported retainer for ceramic FPD**
A ceramic retainer for a fixed partial denture that gains retention, support and stability from an implant.

D6076 **implant supported retainer for FPD – porcelain fused to high noble alloys**
A metal-ceramic retainer for a fixed partial denture that gains retention, support and stability from an implant.

\# **D6098** **implant supported retainer – porcelain fused to predominantly base alloys**
A metal-ceramic retainer for a fixed partial denture that gains retention, support, and stability from an implant.

D6099 **implant supported retainer for FPD – porcelain fused to noble alloys**
A metal-ceramic retainer for a fixed partial denture that gains retention, support, and stability from an implant.

D6120 **implant supported retainer – porcelain fused to titanium and titanium alloys**
A metal-ceramic retainer for a fixed partial denture that gains retention, support, and stability from an implant.

D6077 **implant supported retainer for metal FPD – high noble alloys**
A metal retainer for a fixed partial denture that gains retention, support and stability from an implant.

D6121 **implant supported retainer for metal FPD – predominantly base alloys**
A metal retainer for a fixed partial denture that gains retention, support, and stability from an implant.

D6122 **implant supported retainer for metal FPD – noble alloys**
A metal retainer for a fixed partial denture that gains retention, support, and stability from an implant.

D6123 **implant supported retainer for metal FPD – titanium and titanium alloys**
A metal retainer for a fixed partial denture that gains retention, support, and stability from an implant.

Other Implant Services

D6080 **implant maintenance procedures when prostheses are removed and reinserted, including cleansing of prostheses and abutments**
This procedure includes active debriding of the implant(s) and examination of all aspects of the implant system(s), including the occlusion and stability of the superstructure. The patient is also instructed in thorough daily cleansing of the implant(s). This is not a per implant code, and is indicated for implant supported fixed prostheses.

D6081 **scaling and debridement in the presence of inflammation or mucositis of a single implant, including cleaning of the implant surfaces, without flap entry and closure**
This procedure is not performed in conjunction with D1110, D4910, or D4346.

D6085 **provisional implant crown**
Used when a period of healing is necessary prior to fabrication and placement of permanent prosthetic.

D6090 **repair implant supported prosthesis, by report**
This procedure involves the repair or replacement of any part of the implant supported prosthesis.

▲ **D6091** **replacement of replaceable part of semi-precision or precision attachment (male or female component) of implant/abutment supported prosthesis, per attachment**

D6092 **re-cement or re-bond implant/abutment supported crown**

D6093 **re-cement or re-bond implant/abutment supported fixed partial denture**

D6095 **repair implant abutment, by report**
This procedure involves the repair or replacement of any part of the implant abutment.

D6096 **remove broken implant retaining screw**

D6199 **unspecified implant procedure, by report**
Use for a procedure that is not adequately described by a code. Describe the procedure.

D6200–D6999 IX. Prosthodontics, fixed

Each retainer and each pontic constitutes a unit in a fixed partial denture.

Local anesthesia is usually considered to be part of Fixed Prosthodontic procedures.

The term "fixed partial denture" or FPD is synonymous with fixed bridge or bridgework.

Fixed partial denture prosthetic procedures include routine temporary prosthetics. When indicated, interim or provisional codes should be reported separately.

Fixed Partial Denture Pontics

D6205 **pontic – indirect resin based composite**
Not to be used as a temporary or provisional prosthesis.

D6210 **pontic – cast high noble metal**

D6211 **pontic – cast predominantly base metal**

D6212 **pontic – cast noble metal**

D6214 **pontic – titanium and titanium alloys**

D6240 **pontic – porcelain fused to high noble metal**

D6241 **pontic – porcelain fused to predominantly base metal**

D6242 **pontic – porcelain fused to noble metal**

D6243 **pontic – porcelain fused to titanium and titanium alloys**

D6245 **pontic – porcelain/ceramic**

D6250 **pontic – resin with high noble metal**

D6251 **pontic – resin with predominantly base metal**

D6252 **pontic – resin with noble metal**

D6253 **provisional pontic– further treatment or completion of diagnosis necessary prior to final impression**
Not to be used as a temporary pontic for routine prosthetic fixed partial dentures.

Fixed Partial Denture Retainers – Inlays/Onlays

D6545   retainer – cast metal for resin bonded fixed prosthesis

D6548   retainer – porcelain/ceramic for resin bonded fixed prosthesis

D6549   resin retainer – for resin bonded fixed prosthesis

D6600   retainer inlay – porcelain/ceramic, two surfaces

D6601   retainer inlay – porcelain/ceramic, three or more surfaces

D6602   retainer inlay – cast high noble metal, two surfaces

D6603   retainer inlay – cast high noble metal, three or more surfaces

D6604   retainer inlay – cast predominantly base metal, two surfaces

D6605   retainer inlay – cast predominantly base metal, three or more surfaces

D6606   retainer inlay – cast noble metal, two surfaces

D6607   retainer inlay – cast noble metal, three or more surfaces

D6624   retainer inlay – titanium

D6608   retainer onlay – porcelain/ceramic, two surfaces

D6609   retainer onlay – porcelain/ceramic, three or more surfaces

D6610   retainer onlay – cast high noble metal, two surfaces

D6611   retainer onlay – cast high noble metal, three or more surfaces

D6612   retainer onlay – cast predominantly base metal, two surfaces

D6613   retainer onlay – cast predominantly base metal, three or more surfaces

D6614   retainer onlay – cast noble metal, two surfaces

D6615   retainer onlay – cast noble metal, three or more surfaces

D6634   retainer onlay – titanium

Fixed Partial Denture Retainers – Crowns

D6710 retainer crown – indirect resin based composite
Not to be used as a temporary or provisional prosthesis.

D6720 retainer crown – resin with high noble metal

D6721 retainer crown – resin with predominantly base metal

D6722 retainer crown – resin with noble metal

D6740 retainer crown – porcelain/ceramic

D6750 retainer crown – porcelain fused to high noble metal

D6751 retainer crown – porcelain fused to predominantly base metal

D6752 retainer crown – porcelain fused to noble metal

D6753 retainer crown – porcelain fused to titanium and titanium alloys

D6780 retainer crown – ¾ cast high noble metal

D6781 retainer crown – ¾ cast predominantly base metal

D6782 retainer crown – ¾ cast noble metal

D6783 retainer crown – ¾ porcelain/ceramic

D6784 retainer crown ¾ – titanium and titanium alloys

D6790 retainer crown – full cast high noble metal

D6791 retainer crown – full cast predominantly base metal

D6792 retainer crown – full cast noble metal

D6794 retainer crown – titanium and titanium alloys

D6793 provisional retainer crown– further treatment or completion of diagnosis necessary prior to final impression
Not to be used as a temporary retainer crown for routine prosthetic fixed partial dentures.

Other Fixed Partial Denture Services

D6920 **connector bar**
A device attached to fixed partial denture retainer or coping which serves to stabilize and anchor a removable overdenture prosthesis.

D6930 **re-cement or re-bond fixed partial denture**

D6940 **stress breaker**
A non-rigid connector.

D6950 **precision attachment**
A male and female pair constitutes one precision attachment, and is separate from the prosthesis.

D6980 **fixed partial denture repair necessitated by restorative material failure**

D6985 **pediatric partial denture, fixed**
This prosthesis is used primarily for aesthetic purposes.

D6999 **unspecified fixed prosthodontic procedure, by report**
Used for a procedure that is not adequately described by a code. Describe the procedure.

D7000–D7999 X. Oral & Maxillofacial Surgery

Local anesthesia is usually considered to be part of Oral and Maxillofacial Surgical procedures.

For dental benefit reporting purposes a quadrant is defined as four or more contiguous teeth and/or teeth spaces distal to the midline.

Extractions (Includes Local Anesthesia, Suturing If Needed, and Routine Postoperative Care)

D7111   **extraction, coronal remnants – primary tooth**
Removal of soft tissue-retained coronal remnants.

D7140   **extraction, erupted tooth or exposed root (elevation and/or forceps removal)**
Includes removal of tooth structure, minor smoothing of socket bone, and closure, as necessary.

D7210   **extraction, erupted tooth requiring removal of bone and/or sectioning of tooth, and including elevation of mucoperiosteal flap if indicated**
Includes related cutting of gingiva and bone, removal of tooth structure, minor smoothing of socket bone and closure.

D7220   **removal of impacted tooth – soft tissue**
Occlusal surface of tooth covered by soft tissue; requires mucoperiosteal flap elevation.

D7230   **removal of impacted tooth – partially bony**
Part of crown covered by bone; requires mucoperiosteal flap elevation and bone removal.

D7240   **removal of impacted tooth – completely bony**
Most or all of crown covered by bone; requires mucoperiosteal flap elevation and bone removal.

D7241   **removal of impacted tooth – completely bony, with unusual surgical complications**
Most or all of crown covered by bone; unusually difficult or complicated due to factors such as nerve dissection required, separate closure of maxillary sinus required or aberrant tooth position.

   | ● new procedure code   ▲ revision to a nomenclature or descriptor   # Editorial

D7250 **removal of residual tooth roots (cutting procedure)**
Includes cutting of soft tissue and bone, removal of tooth structure, and closure.

D7251 **coronectomy – intentional partial tooth removal**
Intentional partial tooth removal is performed when a neurovascular complication is likely if the entire impacted tooth is removed.

Other Surgical Procedures

D7260 **oroantral fistula closure**
Excision of fistulous tract between maxillary sinus and oral cavity and closure by advancement flap.

D7261 **primary closure of a sinus perforation**
Subsequent to surgical removal of tooth, exposure of sinus requiring repair, or immediate closure of oroantral or oralnasal communication in absence of fistulous tract.

D7270 **tooth re-implantation and/or stabilization of accidentally evulsed or displaced tooth**
Includes splinting and/or stabilization.

D7272 **tooth transplantation (includes re-implantation from one site to another and splinting and/or stabilization)**

D7280 **exposure of an unerupted tooth**
An incision is made and the tissue is reflected and bone removed as necessary to expose the crown of an impacted tooth not intended to be extracted.

D7282 **mobilization of erupted or malpositioned tooth to aid eruption**
To move/luxate teeth to eliminate ankylosis; not in conjunction with an extraction.

D7283 **placement of device to facilitate eruption of impacted tooth**
Placement of an attachment on an unerupted tooth, after its exposure, to aid in its eruption. Report the surgical exposure separately using D7280.

D7285 **incisional biopsy of oral tissue – hard (bone, tooth)**
For partial removal of specimen only. This procedure involves biopsy of osseous lesions and is not used for apicoectomy/periradicular surgery. This procedure does not entail an excision.

D7286 **incisional biopsy of oral tissue – soft**
For partial removal of an architecturally intact specimen only. This procedure is not used at the same time as codes for apicoectomy/periradicular curettage. This procedure does not entail an excision.

D7287 **exfoliative cytological sample collection**
For collection of non-transepithelial cytology sample via mild scraping of the oral mucosa.

D7288 **brush biopsy – transepithelial sample collection**
For collection of oral disaggregated transepithelial cells via rotational brushing of the oral mucosa.

D7290 **surgical repositioning of teeth**
Grafting procedure(s) is/are additional.

D7291 **transseptal fiberotomy/supra crestal fiberotomy, by report**
The supraosseous connective tissue attachment is surgically severed around the involved teeth. Where there are adjacent teeth, the transseptal fiberotomy of a single tooth will involve a minimum of three teeth. Since the incisions are within the gingival sulcus and tissue and the root surface is not instrumented, this procedure heals by the reunion of connective tissue with the root surface on which viable periodontal tissue is present (reattachment).

D7292 **placement of temporary anchorage device [screw retained plate] requiring flap; includes device removal**

D7293 **placement of temporary anchorage device requiring flap; includes device removal**

D7294 **placement of temporary anchorage device without flap; includes device removal**

D7295 **harvest of bone for use in autogenous grafting procedure**
Reported in addition to those autogenous graft placement procedures that do not include harvesting of bone.

D7296 **corticotomy – one to three teeth or tooth spaces, per quadrant**
This procedure involves creating multiple cuts, perforations, or removal of cortical, alveolar or basal bone of the jaw for the purpose of facilitating orthodontic repositioning of the dentition. This procedure includes flap entry and closure. Graft material and membrane, if used, should be reported separately.

D7297 **corticotomy – four or more teeth or tooth spaces, per quadrant**
This procedure involves creating multiple cuts, perforations, or removal of cortical, alveolar or basal bone of the jaw for the purpose of facilitating orthodontic repositioning of the dentition. This procedure includes flap entry and closure. Graft material and membrane, if used, should be reported separately.

Alveoloplasty – Preparation of Ridge

D7310 **alveoloplasty in conjunction with extractions – four or more teeth or tooth spaces, per quadrant**
The alveoloplasty is distinct (separate procedure) from extractions. Usually in preparation for a prosthesis or other treatments such as radiation therapy and transplant surgery.

D7311 **alveoloplasty in conjunction with extractions – one to three teeth or tooth spaces, per quadrant**
The alveoloplasty is distinct (separate procedure) from extractions. Usually in preparation for a prosthesis or other treatments such as radiation therapy and transplant surgery.

D7320 **alveoloplasty not in conjunction with extractions – four or more teeth or tooth spaces, per quadrant**
No extractions performed in an edentulous area. See D7310 if teeth are being extracted concurrently with the alveoloplasty. Usually in preparation for a prosthesis or other treatments such as radiation therapy and transplant surgery.

D7321 **alveoloplasty not in conjunction with extractions – one to three teeth or tooth spaces, per quadrant**
No extractions performed in an edentulous area. See D7311 if teeth are being extracted concurrently with the alveoloplasty. Usually in preparation for a prosthesis or other treatments such as radiation therapy and transplant surgery.

Vestibuloplasty

Any of a series of surgical procedures designed to increase relative alveolar ridge height.

D7340 **vestibuloplasty – ridge extension (secondary epithelialization)**

D7350 **vestibuloplasty – ridge extension (including soft tissue grafts, muscle reattachment, revision of soft tissue attachment and management of hypertrophied and hyperplastic tissue)**

Excision of Soft Tissue Lesions

Includes non-odontogenic cysts.

D7410 **excision of benign lesion up to 1.25 cm**

D7411 **excision of benign lesion greater than 1.25 cm**

D7412 **excision of benign lesion, complicated**
Requires extensive undermining with advancement or rotational flap closure.

D7413 **excision of malignant lesion up to 1.25 cm**

D7414 **excision of malignant lesion greater than 1.25 cm**

D7415 **excision of malignant lesion, complicated**
Requires extensive undermining with advancement or rotational flap closure.

D7465 **destruction of lesion(s) by physical or chemical method, by report**
Examples include using cryo, laser or electro surgery.

Excision of Intra-Osseous Lesions

D7440 **excision of malignant tumor – lesion diameter up to 1.25 cm**

D7441 **excision of malignant tumor – lesion diameter greater than 1.25 cm**

D7450 **removal of benign odontogenic cyst or tumor – lesion diameter up to 1.25 cm**

D7451 **removal of benign odontogenic cyst or tumor – lesion diameter greater than 1.25 cm**

D7460 **removal of benign nonodontogenic cyst or tumor – lesion diameter up to 1.25 cm**

D7461 **removal of benign nonodontogenic cyst or tumor – lesion diameter greater than 1.25 cm**

Excision of Bone Tissue

D7471   **removal of lateral exostosis (maxilla or mandible)**

D7472   **removal of torus palatinus**

D7473   **removal of torus mandibularis**

D7485   **reduction of osseous tuberosity**

D7490   **radical resection of maxilla or mandible**
Partial resection of maxilla or mandible; removal of lesion and defect with margin of normal appearing bone. Reconstruction and bone grafts should be reported separately.

Surgical Incision

D7510   **incision and drainage of abscess – intraoral soft tissue**
Involves incision through mucosa, including periodontal origins.

D7511   **incision and drainage of abscess – intraoral soft tissue – complicated (includes drainage of multiple fascial spaces)**
Incision is made intraorally and dissection is extended into adjacent fascial space(s) to provide adequate drainage of abscess/cellulitis.

D7520   **incision and drainage of abscess – extraoral soft tissue**
Involves incision through skin.

D7521   **incision and drainage of abscess – extraoral soft tissue – complicated (includes drainage of multiple fascial spaces)**
Incision is made extraorally and dissection is extended into adjacent fascial space(s) to provide adequate drainage of abscess/cellulitis.

D7530   **removal of foreign body from mucosa, skin, or subcutaneous alveolar tissue**

D7540   **removal of reaction producing foreign bodies, musculoskeletal system**
May include, but is not limited to, removal of splinters, pieces of wire, etc., from muscle and/or bone.

D7550   **partial ostectomy/sequestrectomy for removal of non-vital bone**
Removal of loose or sloughed-off dead bone caused by infection or reduced blood supply.

D7560   **maxillary sinusotomy for removal of tooth fragment or foreign body**

Treatment of Closed Fractures

D7610   **maxilla – open reduction (teeth immobilized, if present)**
Teeth may be wired, banded or splinted together to prevent movement. Incision required for interosseous fixation.

D7620   **maxilla – closed reduction (teeth immobilized, if present)**
No incision required to reduce fracture. See D7610 if interosseous fixation is applied.

D7630   **mandible – open reduction (teeth immobilized, if present)**
Teeth may be wired, banded or splinted together to prevent movement. Incision required to reduce fracture.

D7640   **mandible – closed reduction (teeth immobilized, if present)**
No incision required to reduce fracture. See D7630 if interosseous fixation is applied.

D7650   **malar and/or zygomatic arch – open reduction**

D7660   **malar and/or zygomatic arch – closed reduction**

D7670   **alveolus – closed reduction, may include stabilization of teeth**
Teeth may be wired, banded or splinted together to prevent movement.

D7671   **alveolus – open reduction, may include stabilization of teeth**
Teeth may be wired, banded or splinted together to prevent movement.

D7680   **facial bones – complicated reduction with fixation and multiple surgical approaches**
Facial bones include upper and lower jaw, cheek, and bones around eyes, nose, and ears.

Treatment of Open Fractures

D7710   **maxilla – open reduction**
Incision required to reduce fracture.

D7720   **maxilla – closed reduction**

D7730   **mandible – open reduction**
Incision required to reduce fracture.

D7740   **mandible – closed reduction**

D7750   **malar and/or zygomatic arch – open reduction**
Incision required to reduce fracture.

D7760   **malar and/or zygomatic arch – closed reduction**

D7770 alveolus – open reduction stabilization of teeth
Fractured bone(s) are exposed to mouth or outside the face.
Incision required to reduce fracture.

D7771 alveolus, closed reduction stabilization of teeth
Fractured bone(s) are exposed to mouth or outside the face.

D7780 facial bones – complicated reduction with fixation and multiple approaches
Incision required to reduce fracture. Facial bones include upper and lower jaw, cheek, and bones around eyes, nose, and ears.

Reduction of Dislocation and Management of Other Temporomandibular Joint Dysfunctions

Procedures that are an integral part of a primary procedure should not be reported separately.

D7810 open reduction of dislocation
Access to TMJ via surgical opening.

D7820 closed reduction of dislocation
Joint manipulated into place; no surgical exposure.

D7830 manipulation under anesthesia
Usually done under general anesthesia or intravenous sedation.

D7840 condylectomy
Removal of all or portion of the mandibular condyle (separate procedure).

D7850 surgical discectomy, with/without implant
Excision of the intra-articular disc of a joint.

D7852 disc repair
Repositioning and/or sculpting of disc; repair of perforated posterior attachment.

D7854 synovectomy
Excision of a portion or all of the synovial membrane of a joint.

D7856 myotomy
Cutting of muscle for therapeutic purposes (separate procedure).

D7858 joint reconstruction
Reconstruction of osseous components including or excluding soft tissues of the joint with autogenous, homologous, or alloplastic materials.

D7860 **arthrotomy**
Cutting into joint (separate procedure).

D7865 **arthroplasty**
Reduction of osseous components of the joint to create a pseudoarthrosis or eliminate an irregular remodeling pattern (osteophytes).

D7870 **arthrocentesis**
Withdrawal of fluid from a joint space by aspiration.

D7871 **non-arthroscopic lysis and lavage**
Inflow and outflow catheters are placed into the joint space. The joint is lavaged and manipulated as indicated in an effort to release minor adhesions and synovial vacuum phenomenon as well as to remove inflammation products from the joint space.

D7872 **arthroscopy – diagnosis, with or without biopsy**

D7873 **arthroscopy: lavage and lysis of adhesions**
Removal of adhesions using the arthroscope and lavage of the joint cavities.

D7874 **arthroscopy: disc repositioning and stabilization**
Repositioning and stabilization of disc using arthroscopic techniques.

D7875 **arthroscopy: synovectomy**
Removal of inflamed and hyperplastic synovium (partial/complete) via an arthroscopic technique.

D7876 **arthroscopy: discectomy**
Removal of disc and remodeled posterior attachment via the arthroscope.

D7877 **arthroscopy: debridement**
Removal of pathologic hard and/or soft tissue using the arthroscope.

D7880 **occlusal orthotic device, by report**
Presently includes splints provided for treatment of temporomandibular joint dysfunction.

D7881 **occlusal orthotic device adjustment**

D7899 **unspecified TMD therapy, by report**
Used for procedure that is not adequately described by a code. Describe procedure.

Repair of Traumatic Wounds

Excludes closure of surgical incisions.

D7910 **suture of recent small wounds up to 5 cm**

Complicated Suturing (Reconstruction Requiring Delicate Handling of Tissues and Wide Undermining for Meticulous Closure)

Excludes closure of surgical incisions.

D7911 **complicated suture – up to 5 cm**

D7912 **complicated suture – greater than 5 cm**

Other Repair Procedures

D7920 **skin graft (identify defect covered, location and type of graft)**

D7921 **collection and application of autologous blood concentrate product**

D7922 **placement of intra-socket biological dressing to aid in hemostasis or clot stabilization, per site**
This procedure can be performed at time and/or after extraction to aid in hemostasis. The socket is packed with a hemostatic agent to aid in hemostasis and or clot stabilization.

D7940 **osteoplasty – for orthognathic deformities**
Reconstruction of jaws for correction of congenital, developmental or acquired traumatic or surgical deformity.

D7941 **osteotomy – mandibular rami**

D7943 **osteotomy – mandibular rami with bone graft; includes obtaining the graft**

D7944 **osteotomy – segmented or subapical**
Report by range of tooth numbers within segment.

D7945 **osteotomy – body of mandible**
Sectioning of lower jaw. This includes the exposure, bone cut, fixation, routine wound closure and normal post-operative follow-up care.

D7946 **LeFort I (maxilla – total)**
Sectioning of the upper jaw. This includes exposure, bone cuts, downfracture, repositioning, fixation, routine wound closure and normal post-operative follow-up care.

D7947 **LeFort I (maxilla – segmented)**
When reporting a surgically assisted palatal expansion without downfracture, this code would entail a reduced service and should be "by report."

D7948 **LeFort II or LeFort III (osteoplasty of facial bones for midface hypoplasia or retrusion) – without bone graft**
Sectioning of upper jaw. This includes exposure, bone cuts, downfracture, segmentation of maxilla, repositioning, fixation, routine wound closure and normal post-operative follow-up care.

D7949 **LeFort II or LeFort III – with bone graft**
Includes obtaining autografts.

D7950 **osseous, osteoperiosteal, or cartilage graft of the mandible or maxilla – autogenous or nonautogenous, by report**
This procedure is for ridge augmentation or reconstruction to increase height, width and/or volume of residual alveolar ridge. It includes obtaining graft material. Placement of a barrier membrane, if used, should be reported separately.

D7951 **sinus augmentation with bone or bone substitutes via a lateral open approach**
The augmentation of the sinus cavity to increase alveolar height for reconstruction of edentulous portions of the maxilla. This procedure is performed via a lateral open approach. This includes obtaining the bone or bone substitutes. Placement of a barrier membrane if used should be reported separately.

D7952 **sinus augmentation via a vertical approach**
The augmentation of the sinus to increase alveolar height by vertical access through the ridge crest by raising the floor of the sinus and grafting as necessary. This includes obtaining the bone or bone substitutes.

D7953 **bone replacement graft for ridge preservation – per site**
Graft is placed in an extraction or implant removal site at the time of the extraction or removal to preserve ridge integrity (e.g., clinically indicated in preparation for implant reconstruction or where alveolar contour is critical to planned prosthetic reconstruction). Does not include obtaining graft material. Membrane, if used should be reported separately.

D7955 **repair of maxillofacial soft and/or hard tissue defect**
Reconstruction of surgical, traumatic, or congenital defects of the facial bones, including the mandible, may utilize graft materials in conjunction with soft tissue procedures to repair and restore the facial bones to form and function. This does not include obtaining the graft and these procedures may require multiple surgical approaches. This procedure does not include edentulous maxilla and mandibular reconstruction for prosthetic considerations.

● **D7961** **buccal / labial frenectomy (frenulectomy)**

● **D7962** **lingual frenectomy (frenulectomy)**

D7963 **frenuloplasty**
Excision of frenum with accompanying excision or repositioning of aberrant muscle and z-plasty or other local flap closure.

D7970 **excision of hyperplastic tissue – per arch**

D7971 **excision of pericoronal gingiva**
Removal of inflammatory or hypertrophied tissues surrounding partially erupted/impacted teeth.

D7972 **surgical reduction of fibrous tuberosity**

D7979 **non – surgical sialolithotomy**
A sialolith is removed from the gland or ductal portion of the gland without surgical incision into the gland or the duct of the gland; for example via manual manipulation, ductal dilation, or any other non-surgical method.

D7980 **surgical sialolithotomy**
Procedure by which a stone within a salivary gland or its duct is removed, either intraorally or extraorally.

D7981 **excision of salivary gland, by report**

D7982 **sialodochoplasty**
Procedure for the repair of a defect and/or restoration of a portion of a salivary gland duct.

D7983 **closure of salivary fistula**
Closure of an opening between a salivary duct and/or gland and the cutaneous surface, or an opening into the oral cavity through other than the normal anatomic pathway.

D7990 **emergency tracheotomy**
Formation of a tracheal opening usually below the cricoid cartilage to allow for respiratory exchange.

D7991 **coronoidectomy**
Removal of the coronoid process of the mandible.

● **D7993** **surgical placement of craniofacial implant – extra oral**
Surgical placement of a craniofacial implant to aid in retention of an auricular, nasal, or orbital prosthesis.

● **D7994** **surgical placement: zygomatic implant**
An implant placed in the zygomatic bone and exiting through the maxillary mucosal tissue providing support and attachment of a maxillary dental prosthesis.

D7995 **synthetic graft – mandible or facial bones, by report**
Includes allogenic material.

D7996 **implant-mandible for augmentation purposes (excluding alveolar ridge), by report**

D7997 **appliance removal (not by dentist who placed appliance), includes removal of archbar**

D7998 **intraoral placement of a fixation device not in conjunction with a fracture**
The placement of intermaxillary fixation appliance for documented medically accepted treatments not in association with fractures.

D7999 **unspecified oral surgery procedure, by report**
Used for a procedure that is not adequately described by a code. Describe the procedure.

D8000–D8999 XI. Orthodontics

Dentition

Primary Dentition: Teeth developed and erupted first in order of time.

Transitional Dentition: The final phase of the transition from primary to adult teeth, in which the deciduous molars and canines are in the process of shedding and the permanent successors are emerging.

Adolescent Dentition: The dentition that is present after the normal loss of primary teeth and prior to cessation of growth that would affect orthodontic treatment.

Adult Dentition: The dentition that is present after the cessation of growth that would affect orthodontic treatment.

All of the following orthodontic treatment codes may be used more than once for the treatment of a particular patient depending on the particular circumstance. A patient may require more than one interceptive procedure or more than one limited procedure depending on their particular problem.

Limited Orthodontic Treatment

Orthodontic treatment with a limited objective, not necessarily involving the entire dentition. It may be directed at the only existing problem, or at only one aspect of a larger problem in which a decision is made to defer or forego more comprehensive therapy.

D8010 **limited orthodontic treatment of the primary dentition**

D8020 **limited orthodontic treatment of the transitional dentition**

D8030 **limited orthodontic treatment of the adolescent dentition**

D8040 **limited orthodontic treatment of the adult dentition**

Interceptive Orthodontic Treatment

Interceptive orthodontics is an extension of preventive orthodontics that may include localized tooth movement. Such treatment may occur in the primary or transitional dentition and may include such procedures as the redirection of ectopically erupting teeth, correction of dental crossbite or recovery of space loss where overall space is inadequate. When initiated during the incipient stages of a developing problem, interceptive orthodontics may reduce the severity of the malformation and mitigate its cause. Complicating factors such as skeletal disharmonies, overall space deficiency, or other conditions may require subsequent comprehensive therapy.

D8050   interceptive orthodontic treatment of the primary dentition

D8060   interceptive orthodontic treatment of the transitional dentition

Comprehensive Orthodontic Treatment

Comprehensive orthodontic care includes a coordinated diagnosis and treatment leading to the improvement of a patient's craniofacial dysfunction and/or dentofacial deformity which may include anatomical, functional and/or aesthetic relationships. Treatment may utilize fixed and/or removable orthodontic appliances and may also include functional and/or orthopedic appliances in growing and non-growing patients. Adjunctive procedures to facilitate care may be required. Comprehensive orthodontics may incorporate treatment phases focusing on specific objectives at various stages of dentofacial development.

D8070   comprehensive orthodontic treatment of the transitional dentition

D8080   comprehensive orthodontic treatment of the adolescent dentition

D8090   comprehensive orthodontic treatment of the adult dentition

Minor Treatment to Control Harmful Habits

D8210   **removable appliance therapy**
Removable indicates patient can remove; includes appliances for thumb sucking and tongue thrusting.

D8220   **fixed appliance therapy**
Fixed indicates patient cannot remove appliance; includes appliances for thumb sucking and tongue thrusting.

Other Orthodontic Services

D8660   **pre-orthodontic treatment examination to monitor growth and development**
Periodic observation of patient dentition, at intervals established by the dentist, to determine when orthodontic treatment should begin. Diagnostic procedures are documented separately.

D8670   **periodic orthodontic treatment visit**

D8680   **orthodontic retention (removal of appliances, construction and placement of retainer(s))**

D8681   **removable orthodontic retainer adjustment**

D8690   **orthodontic treatment (alternative billing to a contract fee)**
Services provided by dentist other than original treating dentist. A method of payment between the provider and responsible party for services that reflect an open-ended fee arrangement.

D8695   **removal of fixed orthodontic appliances for reasons other than completion of treatment**

D8696   **repair of orthodontic appliance – maxillary**
Does not include bracket and standard fixed orthodontic appliances. It does include functional appliances and palatal expanders.

D8697   **repair of orthodontic appliance – mandibular**
Does not include bracket and standard fixed orthodontic appliances. It does include functional appliances and palatal expanders.

D8698   **re-cement or re-bond fixed retainer – maxillary**

D8699   **re-cement or re-bond fixed retainer – mandibular**

D8701	repair of fixed retainer, includes reattachment – maxillary
D8702	repair of fixed retainer, includes reattachment – mandibular
D8703	replacement of lost or broken retainer – maxillary
D8704	replacement of lost or broken retainer – mandibular

D8999 **unspecified orthodontic procedure, by report**
Used for a procedure that is not adequately described by a code. Describe the procedure.

D9000–D9999 XII. Adjunctive General Services

Unclassified Treatment

D9110 **palliative (emergency) treatment of dental pain – minor procedure**
This is typically reported on a "per visit" basis for emergency treatment of dental pain.

D9120 **fixed partial denture sectioning**
Separation of one or more connections between abutments and/or pontics when some portion of a fixed prosthesis is to remain intact and serviceable following sectioning and extraction or other treatment. Includes all recontouring and polishing of retained portions.

D9130 **temporomandibular joint dysfunction – non-invasive physical therapies**
Therapy including but not limited to massage, diathermy, ultrasound, or cold application to provide relief from muscle spasms, inflammation or pain, intending to improve freedom of motion and joint function. This should be reported on a per session basis.

Anesthesia

D9210 **local anesthesia not in conjunction with operative or surgical procedures**

D9211 **regional block anesthesia**

D9212 **trigeminal division block anesthesia**

D9215 **local anesthesia in conjunction with operative or surgical procedures**

D9219 **evaluation for moderate sedation, deep sedation or general anesthesia**

D9222 **deep sedation/general anesthesia – first 15 minutes**
Anesthesia time begins when the doctor administering the anesthetic agent initiates the appropriate anesthesia and non-invasive monitoring protocol and remains in continuous attendance of the patient. Anesthesia services are considered completed when the patient may be safely left under the observation of trained personnel and the doctor may safely leave the room to attend to other patients or duties.

The level of anesthesia is determined by the anesthesia provider's documentation of the anesthetic effects upon the central nervous system and not dependent upon the route of administration.

D9223 **deep sedation/general anesthesia – each subsequent 15 minute increment**

D9230 **inhalation of nitrous oxide/analgesia, anxiolysis**

D9239 **intravenous moderate (conscious) sedation/analgesia – first 15 minutes**
Anesthesia time begins when the doctor administering the anesthetic agent initiates the appropriate anesthesia and non-invasive monitoring protocol and remains in continuous attendance of the patient. Anesthesia services are considered completed when the patient may be safely left under the observation of trained personnel and the doctor may safely leave the room to attend to other patients or duties.

The level of anesthesia is determined by the anesthesia provider's documentation of the anesthetic effects upon the central nervous system and not dependent upon the route of administration.

D9243 **intravenous moderate (conscious) sedation/analgesia – each subsequent 15 minute increment**

D9248 **non-intravenous conscious sedation**
This includes non-IV minimal and moderate sedation.

A medically controlled state of depressed consciousness while maintaining the patient's airway, protective reflexes and the ability to respond to stimulation or verbal commands. It includes non-intravenous administration of sedative and/or analgesic agent(s) and appropriate monitoring.

The level of anesthesia is determined by the anesthesia provider's documentation of the anesthetic's effects upon the central nervous system and not dependent upon the route of administration.

Professional Consultation

D9310 **consultation – diagnostic service provided by dentist or physician other than requesting dentist or physician**
A patient encounter with a practitioner whose opinion or advice regarding evaluation and/or management of a specific problem; may be requested by another practitioner or appropriate source. The consultation includes an oral evaluation. The consulted practitioner may initiate diagnostic and/or therapeutic services.

D9311 **consultation with a medical health care professional**
Treating dentist consults with a medical health care professional concerning medical issues that may affect patient's planned dental treatment.

Professional Visits

D9410 **house/extended care facility call**
Includes visits to nursing homes, long-term care facilities, hospice sites, institutions, etc. Report in addition to reporting appropriate code numbers for actual services performed.

D9420 **hospital or ambulatory surgical center call**
Care provided outside the dentist's office to a patient who is in a hospital or ambulatory surgical center. Services delivered to the patient on the date of service are documented separately using the applicable procedure codes.

D9430 **office visit for observation (during regularly scheduled hours) – no other services performed**

D9440 **office visit – after regularly scheduled hours**

D9450 **case presentation, detailed and extensive treatment planning**
Established patient. Not performed on same day as evaluation.

Drugs

D9610   therapeutic parenteral drug, single administration
Includes single administration of antibiotics, steroids, anti-inflammatory drugs, or other therapeutic medications. This code should not be used to report administration of sedative, anesthetic or reversal agents.

D9612   therapeutic parenteral drugs, two or more administrations, different medications
Includes multiple administrations of antibiotics, steroids, anti-inflammatory drugs or other therapeutic medications. This code should not be used to report administration of sedatives, anesthetic or reversal agents.

This code should be reported when two or more different medications are necessary and should not be reported in addition to code D9610 on the same date.

D9613   infiltration of sustained release therapeutic drug – single or multiple sites
Infiltration of a sustained release pharmacologic agent for long acting surgical site pain control. Not for local anesthesia purposes.

D9630   drugs or medicaments dispensed in the office for home use
Includes, but is not limited to oral antibiotics, oral analgesics, and topical fluoride; does not include writing prescriptions.

Miscellaneous Services

D9910   application of desensitizing medicament
Includes in-office treatment for root sensitivity. Typically reported on a "per visit" basis for application of topical fluoride. This code is not to be used for bases, liners or adhesives used under restorations.

D9911   application of desensitizing resin for cervical and/or root surface, per tooth
Typically reported on a "per tooth" basis for application of adhesive resins. This code is not to be used for bases, liners, or adhesives used under restorations.

D9920   behavior management, by report
May be reported in addition to treatment provided. Should be reported in 15-minute increments.

  | ● new procedure code   ▲ revision to a nomenclature or descriptor # Editorial

D9930 **treatment of complications (post-surgical) – unusual circumstances, by report**
For example, treatment of a dry socket following extraction or removal of bony sequestrum.

D9932 **cleaning and inspection of removable complete denture, maxillary**
This procedure does not include any adjustments.

D9933 **cleaning and inspection of removable complete denture, mandibular**
This procedure does not include any adjustments.

D9934 **cleaning and inspection of removable partial denture, maxillary**
This procedure does not include any adjustments.

D9935 **cleaning and inspection of removable partial denture, mandibular**
This procedure does not include any adjustments.

D9941 **fabrication of athletic mouthguard**

D9942 **repair and/or reline of occlusal guard**

D9943 **occlusal guard adjustment**

D9944 **occlusal guard – hard appliance, full arch**
Removable dental appliance designed to minimize the effects of bruxism or other occlusal factors. Not to be reported for any type of sleep apnea, snoring or TMD appliances.

D9945 **occlusal guard – soft appliance, full arch**
Removable dental appliance designed to minimize the effects of bruxism or other occlusal factors. Not to be reported for any type of sleep apnea, snoring or TMD appliances.

D9946 **occlusal guard – hard appliance, partial arch**
Removable dental appliance designed to minimize the effects of bruxism or other occlusal factors. Provides only partial occlusal coverage such as anterior deprogrammer. Not to be reported for any type of sleep apnea, snoring or TMD appliances.

D9950 **occlusion analysis – mounted case**
Includes, but is not limited to, facebow, interocclusal records tracings, and diagnostic wax-up; for diagnostic casts, see D0470.

D9951   occlusal adjustment – limited
May also be known as equilibration; reshaping the occlusal surfaces of teeth to create harmonious contact relationships between the maxillary and mandibular teeth. Presently includes discing/odontoplasty/enamoplasty. Typically reported on a "per visit" basis. This should not be reported when the procedure only involves bite adjustment in the routine post-delivery care for a direct/indirect restoration or fixed/removable prosthodontics.

D9952   occlusal adjustment – complete
Occlusal adjustment may require several appointments of varying length, and sedation may be necessary to attain adequate relaxation of the musculature. Study casts mounted on an articulating instrument may be utilized for analysis of occlusal disharmony. It is designed to achieve functional relationships and masticatory efficiency in conjunction with restorative treatment, orthodontics, orthognathic surgery, or jaw trauma when indicated. Occlusal adjustment enhances the healing potential of tissues affected by the lesions of occlusal trauma.

D9970   enamel microabrasion
The removal of discolored surface enamel defects resulting from altered mineralization or decalcification of the superficial enamel layer. Submit per treatment visit.

▲ **D9971   odontoplasty – per tooth**
Removal/reshaping of enamel surfaces or projections.

D9972   external bleaching – per arch – performed in office

D9973   external bleaching – per tooth

D9974   internal bleaching – per tooth

D9975   external bleaching for home application, per arch; includes materials and fabrication of custom trays

Non-clinical procedures

D9961   duplicate/copy patient's records

D9985   sales tax

D9986   missed appointment

D9987   cancelled appointment

D9990 **certified translation or sign-language services – per visit**

D9991 **dental case management – addressing appointment compliance barriers**
Individualized efforts to assist a patient to maintain scheduled appointments by solving transportation challenges or other barriers.

D9992 **dental case management – care coordination**
Assisting in a patient's decisions regarding the coordination of oral health care services across multiple providers, provider types, specialty areas of treatment, health care settings, health care organizations and payment systems. This is the additional time and resources expended to provide experience or expertise beyond that possessed by the patient.

D9993 **dental case management – motivational interviewing**
Patient-centered, personalized counseling using methods such as Motivational Interviewing (MI) to identify and modify behaviors interfering with positive oral health outcomes. This is a separate service from traditional nutritional or tobacco counseling.

D9994 **dental case management – patient education to improve oral health literacy**
Individual, customized communication of information to assist the patient in making appropriate health decisions designed to improve oral health literacy, explained in a manner acknowledging economic circumstances and different cultural beliefs, values, attitudes, traditions and language preferences, and adopting information and services to these differences, which requires the expenditure of time and resources beyond that of an oral evaluation or case presentation.

D9997 **dental case management – patients with special health care needs**
Special treatment considerations for patients/individuals with physical, medical, developmental or cognitive conditions resulting in substantial functional limitations, which require that modifications be made to delivery of treatment to provide comprehensive oral health care services.

D9995 **teledentistry – synchronous; real-time encounter**
Reported in addition to other procedures (e.g., diagnostic) delivered to the patient on the date of service.

D9996 **teledentistry – asynchronous; information stored and forwarded to dentist for subsequent review**
Reported in addition to other procedures (e.g., diagnostic) delivered to the patient on the date of service.

D9999 **unspecified adjunctive procedure, by report**
Used for a procedure that is not adequately described by a code. Describe the procedure.

 ● new procedure code ▲ revision to a nomenclature or descriptor # Editorial

Section 2
CDT Code Changes Mark-Up

This CDT Code version is effective January 1, 2021 through December 31, 2021. All changes are illustrated in this section, color-coded as follows:

- Additions will be in blue ink without underlining
- Deletions will be ~~stricken through in red ink~~
- Revisions and Editorial changes will have added text <u>underlined in blue ink</u> and deleted text ~~stricken through in red ink~~.

There are:

- 28 Additions
- 7 Revisions
- 4 Deletions
- 22 Editorial (e.g., syntax; spelling) actions that clarify without changing the CDT Code entry's purpose or scope

As noted in the Preface, the CDT Code is divided into 12 Categories of Service <u>only</u> for the purpose of organization.

Classification of Materials

Additions
None

Revisions
None

Deletions
None

Editorial
None

D0100-D0999 I. Diagnostic

Additions
Eleven (11) codes

D0604 antigen testing for a public health related pathogen, including coronavirus

D0605 antibody testing for a public health related pathogen, including coronavirus

D0701 panoramic radiographic image – image capture only

D0702 2-D cephalometric radiographic image – image capture only

D0703 2-D oral/facial photographic image obtained intra-orally or extra-orally – image capture only

D0704 3-D photographic image – image capture only

D0705 extra-oral posterior dental radiographic image – image capture only
Image limited to exposure of complete posterior teeth in both dental arches. This is a unique image that is not derived from another image.

D0706 intraoral – occlusal radiographic image – image capture only

D0707 intraoral – periapical radiographic image – image capture only

D0708 intraoral – bitewing radiographic image – image capture only
Image axis may be horizontal or vertical.

D0709 intraoral – complete series of radiographic images – image capture only
A radiographic survey of the whole mouth, usually consisting of 14–22 images (periapical and posterior bitewing as indicated) intended to display the crowns and roots of all teeth, periapical areas and alveolar bone.

Revisions
None

Deletions
None

Editorial
Two (2) codes

D0120   **periodic oral evaluation – established patient**
An evaluation performed on a patient of record to determine any changes in the patient's dental and medical health status since a previous comprehensive or periodic evaluation. This includes an oral cancer evaluation ~~and~~, periodontal screening where indicated, and may require interpretation of information acquired through additional diagnostic procedures. Report additional diagnostic procedures separately.

D0150   **comprehensive oral evaluation – new or established patient**
Used by a general dentist and/or a specialist when evaluating a patient comprehensively. This applies to new patients; established patients who have had a significant change in health conditions or other unusual circumstances, by report, or established patients who have been absent from active treatment for three or more years. It is a thorough evaluation and recording of the extraoral and intraoral hard and soft tissues. It may require interpretation of information acquired through additional diagnostic procedures. Additional diagnostic procedures should be reported separately.

This includes an evaluation for oral cancer ~~where indicated,~~ the evaluation and recording of the patient's dental and medical history and a general health assessment. It may include the evaluation and recording of dental caries, missing or unerupted teeth, restorations, existing prostheses, occlusal relationships, periodontal conditions (including periodontal screening and/or charting), hard and soft tissue anomalies, etc.

D1000–D1999 II. Preventive

Additions
Two (2) codes

D1321 **counseling for the control and prevention of adverse oral, behavioral, and systemic health effects associated with high-risk substance use**
Counseling services may include patient education about adverse oral, behavioral, and systemic effects associated with high-risk substance use and administration routes. This includes ingesting, injecting, inhaling and vaping. Substances used in a high-risk manner may include but are not limited to alcohol, opioids, nicotine, cannabis, methamphetamine and other pharmaceuticals or chemicals.

D1355 **caries preventive medicament application – per tooth**
For primary prevention or remineralization. Medicaments applied do not include topical fluorides.

Revisions
Four (4) codes

D1110 **prophylaxis – adult**
Removal of plaque, calculus and stains from tooth structures <u>and implants</u> in the permanent and transitional dentition. It is intended to control local irritational factors.

D1120 **prophylaxis – child**
Removal of plaque, calculus and stains from tooth structures <u>and implants</u> in the primary and transitional dentition. It is intended to control local irritational factors.

D1557 **removal of fixed bilateral space maintainer – maxillary**
~~Procedure performed by dentist or practice that did not originally place the appliance.~~

D1558 **removal of fixed bilateral space maintainer – mandibular**
~~Procedure performed by dentist or practice that did not originally place the appliance.~~

Deletions
None

Editorial
None

D2000–D2999 III. Restorative

Additions
One (1) code

D2928   prefabricated porcelain/ceramic crown – permanent tooth

Revisions
None

Deletions
None

Editorial
Three (3) codes

D2960   labial veneer (resin laminate) – ~~chairside~~ <u>direct</u>
Refers to labial/facial direct resin bonded veneers.

D2961   labial veneer (resin laminate) – ~~laboratory~~ <u>indirect</u>
Refers to labial/facial indirect resin bonded veneers.

D2962   labial veneer (porcelain laminate) – ~~laboratory~~ <u>indirect</u>
Refers also to facial veneers that extend interproximally and/or cover the incisal edge. Porcelain/ceramic veneers presently include all ceramic and porcelain veneers.

D3000–D3999 IV. Endodontics

Additions
Six (6) codes

D3471 **surgical repair of root resorption - anterior**
For surgery on root of anterior tooth. Does not include placement of restoration.

D3472 **surgical repair of root resorption – premolar**
For surgery on root of premolar tooth. Does not include placement of restoration.

D3473 **surgical repair of root resorption – molar**
For surgery on root of molar tooth. Does not include placement of restoration.

D3501 **surgical exposure of root surface without apicoectomy or repair of root resorption – anterior**
Exposure of root surface followed by observation and surgical closure of the exposed area. Not to be used for or in conjunction with apicoectomy or repair of root resorption.

D3502 **surgical exposure of root surface without apicoectomy or repair of root resorption – premolar**
Exposure of root surface followed by observation and surgical closure of the exposed area. Not to be used for or in conjunction with apicoectomy or repair of root resorption.

D3503 **surgical exposure of root surface without apicoectomy or repair of root resorption – molar**
Exposure of root surface followed by observation and surgical closure of the exposed area. Not to be used for or in conjunction with apicoectomy or repair of root resorption.

Revisions
None

Deletions
One (1) code

~~D3427   periradicular surgery without apicoectomy~~

Editorial
None

D4000–D4999 V. Periodontics

Additions
None

Revisions
None

Deletions
None

Editorial
None

D5000–D5899 VI. Prosthodontics, removable

Additions
None

Revisions
None

Deletions
None

Editorial
Sixteen (16) codes

Partial Dentures (Including Routine Post-Delivery Care)

D5225 maxillary partial denture - flexible base (including ~~any clasps,~~ <u>retentive/clasping materials,</u> rests, and teeth)

D5226 mandibular partial denture – flexible base (including ~~any clasps,~~ <u>retentive/clasping materials,</u> rests, and teeth)

D5282 removable unilateral partial denture – one piece cast metal (including ~~clasps~~ <u>retentive/clasping materials,</u> rests, and teeth), maxillary

D5283 removable unilateral partial denture – one piece cast metal (including ~~clasps~~ <u>retentive/clasping materials, rests,</u> and teeth), mandibular

D5284 removable unilateral partial denture – one piece flexible base (including ~~clasps~~ <u>retentive/clasping materials, rests,</u> and teeth) – per quadrant

D5286 removable unilateral partial denture – one piece resin (including ~~clasps~~ <u>retentive/clasping materials, rests,</u> and teeth) – per quadrant

Denture Reline Procedures

D5730 reline complete maxillary denture (~~chairside~~ <u>direct</u>)

D5731 reline complete mandibular denture (~~chairside~~ <u>direct</u>)

D5740 reline maxillary partial denture (~~chairside~~ <u>direct</u>)

D5741   reline mandibular partial denture (~~chairside~~ <u>direct</u>)

D5750   reline complete maxillary denture (~~laboratory~~ <u>indirect</u>)

D5751   reline complete mandibular denture (~~laboratory~~ <u>indirect</u>)

D5760   reline maxillary partial denture (~~laboratory~~ <u>indirect</u>)

D5761   reline mandibular partial denture (~~laboratory~~ <u>indirect</u>)

Interim Prosthesis

D5820   interim partial denture ~~(maxillary)~~ <u>(including retentive/clasping materials, rests, and teeth), maxillary</u>
~~Includes any necessary clasps and rests.~~

D5821   interim partial denture ~~(mandibular)~~ <u>(including retentive/clasping materials, rests, and teeth), mandibular</u>
~~Includes any necessary clasps and rests.~~

D5900–D5999 VII. Maxillofacial Prosthetics

Additions
Two (2) codes

D5995 periodontal medicament carrier with peripheral seal – laboratory processed – maxillary
A custom fabricated, laboratory processed carrier for the maxillary arch that covers the teeth and alveolar mucosa. Used as a vehicle to deliver prescribed medicaments for sustained contact with the gingiva, alveolar mucosa, and into the periodontal sulcus or pocket.

D5996 periodontal medicament carrier with peripheral seal – laboratory processed – mandibular
A custom fabricated, laboratory processed carrier for the mandibular arch that covers the teeth and alveolar mucosa. Used as a vehicle to deliver prescribed medicaments for sustained contact with the gingiva, alveolar mucosa, and into the periodontal sulcus or pocket.

Revisions
None

Deletions
One (1) code

~~**D5994 periodontal medicament carrier with peripheral seal– laboratory processed**~~
~~A custom fabricated, laboratory processed carrier that covers the teeth and alveolar mucosa. Used as a vehicle to deliver prescribed medicaments for sustained contact with the gingiva, alveolar mucosa, and into the periodontal sulcus or pocket.~~

Editorial
None

D6000–D6199 VIII. Implant Services

Additions
Two (2) codes

D6191 **semi-precision abutment – placement**
This procedure is the initial placement, or replacement, of a semi-precision abutment on the implant body.

D6192 **semi-precision attachment – placement**
This procedure involves the luting of the initial, or replacement, semi-precision attachment to the removable prosthesis.

Revisions
Two (2) codes

D6011 <u>surgical access to an implant body</u> **(second stage implant surgery)**
~~Surgical access to an implant body for placement of a healing cap or to enable placement of an abutment.~~ This procedure, also known as second stage implant surgery, involves removal of tissue that covers the implant body so that a fixture of any type can be placed, or an existing fixture be replaced with another. Examples of fixtures include but are not limited to healing caps, abutments shaped to help contour the gingival margins or the final restorative prosthesis.

D6091 **replacement of** <u>replaceable part of</u> **semi-precision or precision attachment (male or female component) of implant/abutment supported prosthesis, per attachment**
~~This procedure applies to the replaceable male or female component of the attachment.~~

Deletions
One (1) code

~~**D6052** **semi-precision attachment abutment**~~
~~Includes placement of keeper assembly.~~

Editorial
One (1) code

D6098 **implant supported retainer – porcelain fused to predominantly base alloys**
A metal-ceramic retainer for a fixed partial denture that gains retention, support and stability from an ~~abutment on an~~ implant.

D6200–D6999 IX. Prosthodontics, fixed

Additions
None

Revisions
None

Deletions
None

Editorial
None

D7000–D7999 X. Oral & Maxillofacial Surgery

Additions
Four (4) codes

D7961 **buccal / labial frenectomy (frenulectomy)**

D7962 **lingual frenectomy (frenulectomy)**

D7993 **surgical placement of craniofacial implant – extra oral**
Surgical placement of a craniofacial implant to aid in retention of an auricular, nasal, or orbital prosthesis.

D7994 **surgical placement: zygomatic implant**
An implant placed in the zygomatic bone and exiting through the maxillary mucosal tissue providing support and attachment of a maxillary dental prosthesis.

Revisions
None

Deletions
One (1) code

~~D7960~~ ~~frenulectomy — also known as frenectomy or frenotomy — separate procedure not incidental to another procedure~~
~~Removal or release of mucosal and muscle elements of a buccal, labial or lingual frenum that is associated with a pathological condition, or interferes with proper oral development or treatment.~~

Editorial
None

D8000–D8999 XI. Orthodontics

Additions
None

Revisions
None

Deletions
None

Editorial
None

D9000–D9999 XII. Adjunctive General Services

Additions
None

Revisions
One (1) code

D9971 odontoplasty ~~1–2 teeth; includes removal of enamel projections~~ <ins>–</ins>
<ins>per tooth</ins>
<ins>Removal/reshaping of enamel surfaces or projections.</ins>

Deletions
None

Editorial
None

Section 3

ICD-10-CM Diagnoses for Dental Diseases and Conditions

Table of Contents

ICD-10-CM Preface

Dentists, by virtue of their clinical education, experience, and professional ethics, are the individuals responsible for diagnosis. As such, a dentist is also obligated to select the appropriate diagnosis code for patient records and claim submission.

Both the ADA Dental Claim Form and the HIPAA standard electronic dental claim transaction are able to report up to four diagnosis codes. This capability was added to the claim forms with the expectation that ICD (International Classification of Diseases) would, at some point, become a required data element for dental claim adjudication.

Note: Guidance on reporting ICD codes on dental claims is found in the ADA Dental Claim Form's comprehensive completion instructions. The ICD coding instructions apply to three data items –

    29a – **Diagnosis Code Pointer** ("A" through "D" as applicable from Item 34a)

    34 – **Diagnosis Code List Qualifier** ("AB" for ICD-10-CM)

    34a – **Diagnosis Code(s) / A, B, C, D** (Up to four, with the primary diagnosis adjacent to the letter "A")

These instructions are available online at *ADA.org/en/publications/cdt/ada-dental-claim-form.*

Federal regulations published under the auspices of HIPAA's Administrative Simplification provisions specify only ICD codes as valid on claim submissions.

    Note: There is no immediate and universal mandate to include an ICD-10-CM code on all dental claims. Dental benefit plans are unlikely to establish identical diagnostic code reporting requirements. You should check with each plan for its requirements.

ICD-10-CM became the HIPAA standard on October 1, 2015. It is a code set maintained by the Federal government via an interdepartmental committee comprised of representatives from the Centers for Medicare and Medicaid Services (CMS) and the Centers for Disease Control and Prevention (CDC). Versions are published annually and are effective on October 1st. The complete and current code set is available online at: *www.cms.gov/Medicare/Coding/ICD10.*

    Note: ICD-10-CM does not have a chapter for Dentistry-Only codes. This manual contains a subset of the complete code set, and contains entries identified by ADA member dentists appointed to the Council on Dental Benefit Programs as pertinent to most encounters and services provided to a dentist's patient.

Many diagnoses will be reported using a code from Chapter 12: Diseases of the Digestive System, Oral Cavity and Salivary Glands sub-category (K00-K14). Subcategory (M26) of Chapter 13: Disease of Musculoskeletal Systems offers codes in sub-category M26 that represent dentofacial anomalies Including malocclusion and other disorders of the jaw. The code for a dislocated, fractured or broken tooth is located in Chapter 19: Injury Poisoning and Certain Other Consequences of External Causes. Codes from nearly all sections (A00-Z99) are also included so that findings arising from oral evaluations (e.g., "Z" codes) and relevant clinical information can be captured in the patient's dental record and included on a claim when necessary.

ICD-10-CM codes most applicable to dentistry are listed in this section of the CDT manual. Outside this section's scope are CDT to ICD mappings and medical claim coding. Information on these topics is available in the *CDT Companion* and other offerings in the ADA Catalog.

> **Note**: ICD code guidance herein will assist in selection of appropriate diagnosis codes when a claim for dental services is being filed with the patient's medical benefit plan. Such claims can accommodate up to 12 ICD codes, and reporting requirements are more rigorous than what apply today for claims against dental benefit plans.

Information about the 1500 Health Insurance Claim Form used for claims filed against a patient's medical benefit plan is available online at *www.nucc.org/index. php/1500-claim-form-mainmenu-35*.

ICD code capture is addressed on page 32 of the "1500" form completion instructions.

Introduction

ICD-10-CM codes listed in the following chapters are extracted from the tabular list published by the Centers for Medicare and Medicaid Services (CMS) available online at *www.cms.gov/Medicare/Coding/ICD10*.

CMS also publishes general information on an ICD code's format, and how they are reported on a claim submission. This information, in summary form, follows.

> **Note**: The ICD-10-CM coding information in this section is at an introductory level. It is intended to familiarize dentists and practice staff with the code set, and prompt its use to record diagnostic and descriptive information on patient records and dental claims.

> More specific usage information as ICD-10-CM implementation continues will be contained in future editions. For now such usage information is found in the Tabular List published by CMS referenced above.

ICD Code Format

The ICD-10-CM Tabular List contains categ ories, subcategories and codes, which are combinations of letters, numbers, or both.

- All categories are 3 characters, and a three-character category that has no further subdivision is equivalent to a code.

- Subcategories are either 4 or 5 characters.

- Codes may be 3, 4, 5, 6 or 7 characters; the decimal point is not included in the character count.

- Only complete codes are permissible for reporting, and any applicable 7th character must be assigned.

- Some codes have a placeholder character "X" that is designated for future expansion.

- Some codes have a character that must always be the 7th character in the data field. Codes that have a mandatory 7th character, but not always a 4th, 5th or 6th character, the placeholder "X" must be entered to fill any empty character spaces – e.g., K02.XXX7. An example of a 7th character code with a placeholder "X" would be the initial evaluation of a traumatic fracture of the right upper central incisor S02.5XXA.

General ICD Coding Concepts

An accurate diagnosis, appropriately coded, enables preparation of a treatment plan for necessary dental care that addresses the disease processes and related conditions identified by the dentist.

There are guidelines that a dentist should be aware of when documenting ICD codes in a patient record and on a claim.

1. The first ICD code listed on a patient's dental record and claim for procedures delivered on a specific date of service should be the primary reason for services provided during the office visit.

   a. The second through fourth ICD codes listed are the additional diagnoses applicable to the services provided during the visit.

   b. All ICD codes must clearly document the patient's condition and clinically support the planned and delivered treatment.

   c. Diagnosis information contributes to a robust patient record that supports the dentist's clinical decisions should there be a post-delivery review.

2. Each unique ICD-10-CM diagnosis code may be reported only once for an encounter.

3. An examination with abnormal findings refers to a condition or diagnosis that is newly identified or a change in severity of a chronic condition (e.g., periodontitis) during a routine oral examination.

   a. When assigning a code for "with abnormal findings," additional code(s) should be assigned to identify the specific abnormal finding(s).

4. "Z" codes allow for the description of encounters for routine or preventive examinations; they are not used if the examination is for diagnosis of a suspected condition or for treatment purposes. In such cases the diagnosis code is used.

Presentation Format: Select ICD-10-CM Codes for Dentistry

ICD-10-CM codes and their meanings are presented in 21 separate sections as seen in the Table of Contents. Each of these sections can have one or more chapters where individual ICD codes are listed in ascending alpha-numerical order. These Sections and Chapters reflect the various types of patient encounters and clinical conditions (current and past) that would be considered when treatment planning.

Helpful Hints for ICD-10-CM Coding

Per ICD-10-CM Guidelines, to assign a diagnosis code, the condition has to impact the patient care. "Code all documented conditions that coexist at the time of the encounter/visit and require or affect patient care treatment or management. Do not code conditions that were previously treated and no longer exist. However, history codes (categories Z80-Z87) may be used as secondary codes if the historical condition or family history has an impact on current care or influences treatment."

Users will notice coding guidance within the index and tabular section of ICD-10CM. Some of this information is noted below and will assist the user in assigning the correct diagnosis code.

"Other" Codes – Codes titled "other" or "other specified" are for use when the information in the patient record provides detail for which a specific code does not exist. Alphabetic index entries with NEC in the line designate "other" codes in the tabular list. These alphabetic index entries represent specific disease entities for which no specific code exists so the term is included within an "other" code.

"Unspecified" Codes – Codes titled "unspecified" are for use when the information in the patient record is insufficient to assign a more specific code. For those categories for which an unspecified code is not provided, the "other specified" code may represent both other and unspecified.

Inclusion Terms Note – An "inclusion terms note" is a list of terms included under some codes. These terms are the conditions for which that code is to be used. The terms may be synonyms of the code title, or, in the case of "other specified codes", the terms are a list of the various conditions assigned to that code. The inclusion terms are not necessarily exhaustive. Additional terms found in the Alphabetical Index may also be assigned to a code.

"Code Also" Note – A "code also" note instructs that two codes may be required to fully describe a condition, but this note does not provide sequencing direction. The sequencing depends on the circumstances of the encounter.

"Use Additional Code" Notes – "Use additional code" notes are found in the Tabular List at codes that are not part of an etiology/manifestation pair where a secondary code is useful to fully describe a condition. The sequencing rule is the same as the etiology/manifestation pair, "use additional code" indicates that a secondary code should be added, if known.

Sequela (Late Effects) – A sequela is the residual effect (condition produced) after the acute phase of an illness or injury has terminated. There is no time limit on when a sequela code can be used.

A Note about the Use of Mental Health and Substance Abuse Codes

While several mental health and substance abuse codes have been included in the list below, please assign those diagnoses with care. ICD-10CM codes related to mental health conditions, substance abuse or Human Immunodeficiency Virus (HIV) are protected by the Health Insurance Portability and Accountability Act (HIPAA). Individual state laws may supersede HIPAA when they are more stringent than the federal rules.

Select ICD-10-CM Codes Applicable to Dentistry

1. Dental Encounters

Examinations	
Z01.20	Encounter for dental examination and cleaning without abnormal findings
Z01.21	Encounter for dental examination and cleaning with abnormal findings
Z01.812	Encounter for other preprocedural laboratory examinations
Z01.818	Encounter for other preprocedural examinations
Z01.89	Encounter for other specified special examinations
Z02.6	Encounter for examination for insurance purposes
Z04.1	Encounter for examination and observation following transport accident
Z04.2	Encounter for examination and observation following work accident
Z04.3	Encounter for examination and observation following other accident
Z04.8	Encounter for examination and observation for other specified reasons
Z04.9	Encounter for examination and observation for unspecified reason
Z08	Encounter for follow-up examination after completed treatment for malignant neoplasm
Z09	Encounter for follow-up examination after completed treatment for conditions other than malignant neoplasm
Z12.81	Encounter for screening for malignant neoplasm or oral cavity
Z13.84	Encounter for screening for dental disorders
Z33.1	Pregnant state, incidental
Z41.1	Encounter for cosmetic surgery
Z48.814	Encounter for the surgical aftercare following surgery on the teeth or oral cavity

Preventive Care

Z29.3	Encounter for prophylactic fluoride administration
Z29.8	Encounter for other specified prophylactic measures
Z29.9	Encounter for prophylactic measures, unspecified
Z71.3	Dietary counselling and surveillance
Z71.41	Alcohol counselling and surveillance of alcoholic
Z71.51	Drug abuse counselling and surveillance of drug abuser
Z71.6	Tobacco use and counselling

Post-procedure Complications (Aftercare)

M27.51	Perforation of root canal space due to endodontic treatment
M27.52	Endodontic overfill
M27.59	Other periradicular pathology associated with previous endodontic treatment.
T86.820	Skin graft (allograft) rejection
T86.822	Skin graft (allograft) (autograft) infection — Use additional code to specify infection
T86.828	Other complications of skin graft (allograft) (autograft)
T86.831	Bone graft failure
T86.832	Bone graft infection — Use additional code to specify infection
T86.838	Other complications of bone graft

Post-procedural Aftercare

Z46.3	Encounter for fitting and adjustment of dental prosthetic device
Z46.4	Encounter for fitting and adjustment of orthodontic device
Z48.00	Encounter for change or removal of nonsurgical wound dressing
Z48.01	Encounter for change or removal of surgical wound dressing
Z48.02	Encounter for removal of sutures
Z48.03	Encounter for change or removal of drains
Z48.1	Encounter for planned postprocedural wound closure
Z48.3	Aftercare following surgery for neoplasm
Z48.814	Encounter for surgical aftercare following surgery on the teeth or oral cavity
Z48.89	Encounter for other specified surgical aftercare

Z51.5	Encounter for palliative care
Z51.89	Encounter for other specified aftercare
Z71.2	Person consulting for explanation of examination or test findings
Z53.01	Procedure and treatment not carried out due to patient smoking
Z53.09	Procedure and treatment not carried out because of other contraindication
Z53.1	Procedure and treatment not carried out because of patient's decision for reasons of belief and group pressure
Z53.20	Procedure and treatment not carried out because of patient's decision for unspecified reasons
Z53.21	Procedure and treatment not carried out due to patient leaving prior to being seen by health care provider
Z53.29	Procedure and treatment not carried out because of patient's decision for other reasons
Z53.9	Procedure and treatment not carried out, unspecified reason

2. Dental Caries

Risk Factors

Z91.841	Risk for dental caries, low
Z91.842	Risk for dental caries, moderate
Z91.843	Risk for dental caries, high

Caries

K02.3	Arrested dental caries (decay and cavities) (includes coronal and root caries)
K02.51	Dental caries on pit and fissure surface limited to enamel
K02.52	Dental caries on pit and fissure surface penetrating into dentin
K02.53	Dental caries on pit and fissure surface penetrating into pulp
K02.61	Dental caries on smooth surface limited to enamel
K02.62	Dental caries on smooth surface penetrating into dentin
K02.63	Dental caries on smooth surface penetrating into pulp
K02.7	Dental root caries
K02.9	Dental caries, unspecified

3. Disorders of Teeth

Occlusal Trauma

K08.81	Primary occlusal trauma
K08.82	Secondary occlusal trauma
K08.89	Other specified disorders of teeth and supporting structures (Includes the following — Enlargement of alveolar ridge NOS [not otherwise specified]; Insufficient anatomic crown height, Insufficient clinical crown length; Irregular alveolar process; Toothache NOS)

Tooth Wear

K03.0	Excessive attrition of teeth
K03.1	Abrasion of teeth
K03.2	Erosion of teeth
K03.3	Pathological resorption of teeth

Other Disorders

K03.4	Hypercementosis
K03.5	Ankylosis of teeth
K03.6	Deposits [accretions] on teeth
K03.7	Posteruptive color changes of dental hard tissues
K03.81	Cracked tooth
K03.89	Other specified diseases of hard tissues of teeth
K03.9	Disease of hard tissues of teeth, unspecified

4. Disorders of Pulp and Perapical Tissues

K04.01	Reversible pulpitis
K04.02	Irreversible pulpitis
K04.1	Necrosis of pulp
K04.2	Pulp degeneration
K04.3	Abnormal hard tissue formation in pulp
K04.4	Acute apical periodontitis of pulpal origin
K04.5	Chronic apical periodontitis

K04.6	Periapical abscess with sinus
K04.7	Periapical abscess without sinus
K04.8	Radicular cyst
K04.99	Other diseases of pulp and periapical tissues

5. Diseases and Conditions of the Periodontium

Gingivitis

K05.00	Acute gingivitis, plaque induced
K05.01	Acute gingivitis, non-plaque induced
K05.10	Chronic gingivitis, plaque induced
K05.11	Chronic gingivitis, non-plaque induced

Gingival Recession

K06.011	Localized gingival recession, minimal
K06.012	Localized gingival recession, moderate
K06.013	Localized gingival recession, severe
K06.021	Generalized gingival recession, minimal
K06.022	Generalized gingival recession, moderate
K06.023	Generalized gingival recession, severe

Other Gingival Conditions

K06.1	Gingival enlargement
K06.2	Gingival and edentulous alveolar ridge lesions associated with trauma
K06.3	Horizontal alveolar bone loss
K06.8	Other specified disorders of gingiva and edentulous alveolar ridge

Periodontitis

K05.211	Aggressive periodontitis, localized, slight
K05.212	Aggressive periodontitis, localized, moderate
K05.213	Aggressive periodontitis, localized, severe
K05.221	Aggressive periodontitis, generalized, slight
K05.222	Aggressive periodontitis, generalized, moderate
K05.223	Aggressive periodontitis, generalized, severe

K05.311	Chronic periodontitis, localized, slight
K05.312	Chronic periodontitis, localized, moderate
K05.313	Chronic periodontitis, localized, severe
K05.321	Chronic periodontitis, generalized, slight
K05.322	Chronic periodontitis, generalized, moderate
K05.323	Chronic periodontitis, generalized, severe
K05.4	Periodontosis
K05.5	Other periodontal diseases

6. Alveolar Ridge Disorders

Atrophy of Alveolar Ridge

K08.21	Minimal atrophy of the mandible
K08.22	Moderate atrophy of the mandible
K08.23	Severe atrophy of the mandible
K08.24	Minimal atrophy of maxilla
K08.25	Moderate atrophy of the maxilla
K08.26	Severe atrophy of the maxilla

Alveolar Anomolies

M26.71	Alveolar maxillary hyperplasia
M26.72	Alveolar mandibular hyperplasia
M26.73	Alveolar maxillary hypoplasia
M26.74	Alveolar mandibular hypoplasia
M26.79	Other specified alveolar anomalies

7. Findings of Lost Teeth

Class I: stage of edentulism that is most apt to be successfully treated with complete dentures using conventional prosthodontic techniques.

Class II: characterized by the continued physical degradation of the denture-supporting anatomy. It is also characterized by the early onset of systemic disease interactions and by specific patient management and lifestyle considerations.

Class III: characterized by the need for surgical revision of supporting structures to allow for adequate prosthodontic function.

Class IV: the most debilitating requiring reconstructive surgery when all teeth are missing or the most severely compromised oral manifestations with poor outcome prognosis in partial edentulism. Treatment is primarily prosthodontic in nature with missing teeth or adjacent structures being restored or replaced with artificial, biocompatible structures.

Lost Teeth: Unspecified Causes

K08.101	Complete loss of teeth, unspecified cause, class I
K08.102	Complete loss of teeth, unspecified cause, class II
K08.103	Complete loss of teeth, unspecified cause, class III
K08.104	Complete loss of teeth, unspecified cause, class IV
K08.401	Partial loss of teeth, unspecified cause, class I
K08.402	Partial loss of teeth, unspecified cause, class II
K08.403	Partial loss of teeth, unspecified cause, class III
K08.404	Partial loss of teeth, unspecified cause, class IV

Lost Teeth: Specified Causes

K08.0	Exfoliation of teeth due to systemic causes
K08.191	Complete loss of teeth due to other specified cause, class I
K08.192	Complete loss of teeth due to other specified cause, class II
K08.193	Complete loss of teeth due to other specified cause, class III
K08.194	Complete loss of teeth due to other specified cause, class IV
K08.491	Partial loss of teeth due to other specified cause, class I
K08.492	Partial loss of teeth due to other specified cause, class II
K08.493	Partial loss of teeth due to other specified cause, class III
K08.494	Partial loss of teeth due to other specified cause, class IV

Lost Teeth: Trauma Related

K08.111	Complete loss of teeth due to trauma, class I
K08.112	Complete loss of teeth due to trauma, class II
K08.113	Complete loss of teeth due to trauma, class III
K08.114	Complete loss of teeth due to trauma, class IV
K08.411	Partial loss of teeth due to trauma, class I
K08.412	Partial loss of teeth due to trauma, class II
K08.413	Partial loss of teeth due to trauma, class III
K08.414	Partial loss of teeth due to trauma, class IV

Lost Teeth: Periodontitis Related

K08.121	Complete loss of teeth due to periodontal diseases, class I
K08.122	Complete loss of teeth due to periodontal diseases, class II
K08.123	Complete loss of teeth due to periodontal diseases, class III
K08.124	Complete loss of teeth due to periodontal diseases, class IV
K08.421	Partial loss of teeth due to periodontal diseases, class I
K08.422	Partial loss of teeth due to periodontal diseases, class II
K08.423	Partial loss of teeth due to periodontal diseases, class III
K08.424	Partial loss of teeth due to periodontal diseases, class IV

Lost Teeth: Caries Related

K08.131	Complete loss of teeth due to caries, class I
K08.132	Complete loss of teeth due to caries, class II
K08.133	Complete loss of teeth due to caries, class III
K08.134	Complete loss of teeth due to caries, class IV
K08.431	Partial loss of teeth due to caries, class I
K08.432	Partial loss of teeth due to caries, class II
K08.433	Partial loss of teeth due to caries, class III
K08.434	Partial loss of teeth due to caries, class IV

8. Developmental Disorders of Teeth and Jaws

Number of Teeth

K00.0	Anodontia
K00.1	Supernumerary teeth

Size and Form of Teeth

K00.2	Abnormalities of size and form of teeth
K00.3	Mottled teeth
K00.4	Disturbances in tooth formation
K00.5	Hereditary disturbances in tooth structure, not elsewhere classified
K00.8	Other disorders of tooth development

Tooth Eruption

K00.6	Disturbances in tooth eruption
K00.7	Teething syndrome
K01.0	Embedded teeth
K01.1	Impacted teeth
K08.3	Retained dental root
Z18.32	Retained tooth

Malocclusion

M26.211	Malocclusion, Angle's class I
M26.212	Malocclusion, Angle's class II
M26.213	Malocclusion, Angle's class III
M26.220	Open anterior occlusal relationship
M26.221	Open posterior occlusal relationship
M26.23	Excessive horizontal overlap
M26.24	Reverse articulation
M26.25	Anomalies of interarch distance
M26.29	Other anomalies of dental arch relationship
M26.30	Unspecified anomaly of tooth position of fully erupted tooth or teeth
M26.31	Crowding of fully erupted teeth
M26.32	Excessive spacing of fully erupted teeth
M26.33	Horizontal displacement of fully erupted tooth or teeth

M26.34   Vertical displacement of fully erupted tooth or teeth

M26.35   Rotation of fully erupted tooth or teeth

M26.36   Insufficient interocclusal distance of fully erupted teeth (ridge)

M26.37   Excessive interocclusal distance of fully erupted teeth

M26.39   Other anomalies of tooth position of fully erupted tooth or teeth

M26.51   Abnormal jaw closure

M26.52   Limited mandibular range of motion

M26.53   Deviation in opening and closing of the mandible

M26.54   Insufficient anterior guidance

M26.55   Centric occlusion maximum intercuspation discrepancy

M26.56   Non-working side interference

M26.57   Lack of posterior occlusal support

M26.59   Other dentofacial functional abnormalities

Jaw Anomalies

M26.01   Maxillary hyperplasia

M26.02   Maxillary hypoplasia

M26.03   Mandibular hyperplasia

M26.04   Mandibular hypoplasia

M26.05   Macrogenia

M26.06   Microgenia

M26.07   Excessive tuberosity of jaw

M26.10   Unspecified anomaly of jaw-cranial base relationship

M26.11   Maxillary asymmetry

M26.12   Other jaw asymmetry

M26.19   Other specified anomalies of jaw-cranial base relationship

M26.20   Unspecified anomaly of dental arch relationship

Other Dento-facial Anomalies

M26.81   Anterior soft tissue impingement

M26.82   Posterior soft tissue impingement

M26.89   Other dentofacial anomalies

Cleft Lip and Palate

Q35.1	Cleft hard palate
Q35.3	Cleft soft palate
Q35.5	Cleft hard palate with cleft soft palate
Q35.7	Cleft uvula
Q36.0	Cleft lip, bilateral
Q36.1	Cleft lip, median
Q36.9	Cleft lip, unilateral
Q37.0	Cleft hard palate with bilateral cleft lip
Q37.1	Cleft hard palate with unilateral cleft lip
Q37.2	Cleft soft palate with bilateral cleft lip
Q37.3	Cleft soft palate with unilateral cleft lip
Q37.4	Cleft hard and soft palate with bilateral cleft lip
Q37.5	Cleft hard and soft palate with unilateral cleft lip

Congenital Malformations of Mouth, Tongue and Pharynx

Q38.0	Congenital malformations of lips, not elsewhere classified
Q38.1	Ankyloglossia
Q38.2	Macroglossia
Q38.3	Other congenital malformations of tongue
Q38.4	Congenital malformations of salivary glands and ducts
Q38.5	Congenital malformations of palate, not elsewhere classified
Q38.6	Other congenital malformations of mouth

9. Treatment Complications

Endodontic Complications

M27.51	Perforation of root canal space due to endodontic treatment
M27.52	Endodontic overfill
M27.53	Endodontic underfill
M27.59	Other periradicular pathology associated with previous endodontic treatment

Implant Failure

M27.61	Osseointegration failure of dental implant
M27.62	Post-osseointegration biological failure of dental implant
M27.63	Post-osseointegration mechanical failure of dental implant
M27.69	Other endosseous dental implant failure

Unsatisfactory Restorations

K08.51	Open restoration margins of tooth
K08.52	Unrepairable overhanging of dental restorative materials
K08.530	Fractured dental restorative material without loss of material
K08.531	Fractured dental restorative material with loss of material
K08.54	Contour of existing restoration of tooth biologically incompatible with oral health
K08.55	Allergy to existing dental restorative material
K08.56	Poor aesthetic of existing restoration of tooth
K08.59	Other unsatisfactory restoration of tooth

Complications of Surgical and Medical Care

Note: The appropriate 7th character is to be added to each code that displays an asterisk (*) in the section Complications of Surgical and Medical Care. Insert an "X" as needed as placeholder for unused spaces (e.g., T81.83XA; T81.83XD; T81.83XS).

A = Initial encounter
D = Subsequent encounter
S = Sequela

T81.83X*	Persistent postprocedural fistula
T84.318	Breakdown (mechanical) of other bone devices, implants and grafts
T84.328	Displacement of other bone devices, implants and grafts
T84.398	Other mechanical complication of other bone devices, implants and grafts
T84.59X*	Infection and inflammatory reaction due to other internal joint prosthesis
T85.79X*	Infection and inflammatory reaction due to other internal prosthetic devices, implants and grafts
T88.52X*	Failed moderate sedation during procedure
T88.53X*	Unintended awareness under general anesthesia during procedure
T88.59X*	Other complications of anesthesia
T88.6XX*	Anaphylactic reaction due to adverse effect of correct drug or medicament properly administered

T88.7	Unspecified adverse effect of drug or medicament
T88.8XX*	Other specified complications of surgical and medical care, not elsewhere classified
T88.9	Complication of surgical and medical care, unspecified

Other Post-procedural States

Z98.810	Dental sealant status
Z98.811	Dental restoration status
Z98.818	Other dental procedure status

10. Inflammatory Conditions of the Mucosa

Stomatitis

K12.0	Recurrent oral aphthae
K12.1	Other forms of stomatitis
K12.2	Cellulitis and abscess of mouth
K12.31	Oral mucositis (ulcerative) due to antineoplastic therapy
K12.32	Oral mucositis (ulcerative) due to other drugs
K12.33	Oral mucositis (ulcerative) due to radiation
K12.39	Other oral mucositis (ulcerative)

11. TMJ Diseases and Conditions

TMJ Disorders

M26.601	Right temporomandibular joint disorder, unspecified
M26.602	Left temporomandibular joint disorder, unspecified
M26.603	Bilateral temporomandibular joint disorder, unspecified
M26.609	Unspecified temporomandibular joint disorder, unspecified side
M26.69	Other specified disorders of temporomandibular joint

Adhesions and Ankylosis

M26.611	Adhesions and ankylosis of right temporomandibular joint
M26.612	Adhesions and ankylosis of left temporomandibular joint
M26.613	Adhesions and ankylosis of bilateral temporomandibular joint

Arthralgia

M26.621   Arthralgia of right temporomandibular joint

M26.622   Arthralgia of left temporomandibular joint

M26.623   Arthralgia of bilateral temporomandibular joint

Aricular Disc Disorders

M26.631   Articular disc disorder of right temporomandibular joint

M26.632   Articular disc disorder of left temporomandibular joint

M26.633   Articular disc disorder of bilateral temporomandibular joint

Arthritis of Temporomandibular Joint

M26.641   Arthritis of right temporomandibular joint

M26.642   Arthritis of left temporomandibular joint

M26.643   Arthritis of bilateral temporomandibular joint

Arthropathy of Temporomandibular Joint

M26.651   Arthropathy of right temporomandibular joint

M26.652   Arthropathy of left temporomandibular joint

M26.653   Arthropathy of bilateral temporomandibular joint

12. Breathing, Speech and Sleep Disorders

Mouthbreathing

R06.5   Mouth breathing

R06.83   Snoring

R06.89   Other abnormalities of breathing

Speech

R47.9   Unspecified speech disturbances

F80.89   Other developmental disorders of speech and language

F80.9   Developmental disorder of speech and language, unspecified

Sleep Related Breathing Disorders

G47.30   Sleep apnea, unspecified

G47.31   Primary central sleep apnea

G47.32   High altitude periodic breathing

G47.33   Obstructive sleep apnea (adult) (pediatric)

G47.34   Idiopathic sleep related nonobstructive alveolar hypoventilation

G47.35	Congenital central alveolar hypoventilation syndrome
G47.36	Sleep related hypoventilation in conditions classified elsewhere
G47.37	Central sleep apnea in conditions classified elsewhere
G47.39	Other sleep apnea
G47.63	Sleep related bruxism
G47.8	Other sleep disorders
G47.9	Sleep disorder, unspecified

13. Trauma and Related Conditions

Soft Tissue Injuries

Note: The appropriate 7th character is to be added to each code in this chapter (Soft Tissue Injuries). Insert an "X" as needed as placeholder for unused spaces (e.g., S00.511A; S00.0511D; S00.0511S).

- A = Initial encounter
- D = Subsequent encounter
- S = Sequela

S00.511	Abrasion of lip
S00.512	Abrasion of oral cavity
S00.521	Blister (nonthermal) of lip
S00.522	Blister (nonthermal) of oral cavity
S00.531	Contusion of lip
S00.532	Contusion of oral cavity
S00.541	External constriction of lip
S00.542	External constriction of oral cavity
S01.511	Laceration without foreign body of lip
S01.512	Laceration without foreign body of oral cavity
S01.521	Laceration with foreign body of lip
S01.522	Laceration with foreign body of oral cavity
S01.531	Puncture wound without foreign body of lip
S01.532	Puncture wound without foreign body of oral cavity
S01.541	Puncture wound with foreign body of lip
S01.542	Puncture wound with foreign body of oral cavity
S01.551	Open bite of lip
S01.552	Open bite of oral cavity

Dislocation of Jaw

Note: The appropriate 7th character is to be added to each code in this chapter (Dislocation of Jaw). Insert an "X" as needed as placeholder for unused spaces (e.g., S03.00XA; S03.00XD; S03.00XS).

A = Initial encounter
D = Subsequent encounter
S = Sequela

S03.01X* Dislocation of jaw, right side

S03.02X* Dislocation of jaw, left side

S03.03X* Dislocation of jaw, bilateral

S03.2XX* Dislocation of tooth

S03.41X* Sprain of jaw, right side

S03.42X* Sprain of jaw, left side

S03.43X* Sprain of jaw, bilateral

Fractures: Nasal Bones

Note: The appropriate 7th character is to be added to each code for all "Fractures" which include Nasal bones through Skull and Facial bones. These codes are found in Chapter 19 Injury, Poisoning and Certain Other Consequences of External Causes. Insert an "X" as needed as placeholder for unused spaces (e.g., S02.2XXA; S02.2XXB; S02.2XXD; S02.2XXG; S02.2XXK; S02.2XXS).

A = initial encounter for closed fracture
B = initial encounter for open fracture
D = subsequent encounter for fracture with routine healing
G = subsequent encounter for fracture with delayed healing
K = subsequent encounter for fracture with nonunion
S = sequela

S02.2XX* Fracture of nasal bones

Fractures: Malar

S02.40A Malar fracture, right side

S02.40B Malar fracture, left side

Fractures: Maxilla

S02.40C Maxillary fracture, right side

S02.40D Maxillary fracture, left side

Fractures: Zygoma

S02.40E	Zygomatic fracture, right side
S02.40F	Zygomatic fracture, left side

Fractures: LeFort

S02.411	LeFort I fracture
S02.412	LeFort II fracture
S02.413	LeFort III fracture

Tooth Fractures

S02.5XX*	Fracture of tooth (traumatic)

Fractures: Mandible

S02.601	Fracture of unspecified part of body of right mandible
S02.602	Fracture of unspecified part of body of left mandible
S02.611	Fracture of condylar process of right mandible
S02.612	Fracture of condylar process of left mandible
S02.621	Fracture of subcondylar process of right mandible
S02.622	Fracture of subcondylar process of left mandible
S02.631	Fracture of coronoid process of right mandible
S02.632	Fracture of coronoid process of left mandible
S02.641	Fracture of ramus of right mandible
S02.642	Fracture of ramus of left mandible
S02.651	Fracture of angle of right mandible
S02.652	Fracture of angle of left mandible
S02.66X*	Fracture of symphysis of mandible
S02.69X*	Fracture of mandible of other specified site

Alveolar Fractures

S02.42X*	Fracture of alveolus of maxilla
S02.671	Fracture of alveolus of right mandible
S02.672	Fracture of alveolus of left mandible

Fractures: Skull and Facial Bones

S02.81X*	Fracture of other specified skull and facial bones, right side
S02.82X*	Fracture of other specified skull and facial bones, left side
S02.91	Unspecified fracture of skull
S02.92	Unspecified fracture of facial bones

Foreign Bodies

Note: The appropriate 7th character is to be added to each code in this chapter (Foreign Bodies). Insert an "X" as needed as placeholder for unused spaces (e.g., T17.0XXA; T17.0XXD; T17.0XXS).

- A = Initial encounter
- D = Subsequent encounter
- S = Sequela

T17.0XX*	Foreign body in nasal sinus
S00.551	Superficial foreign body of lip
S00.552	Superficial foreign body of oral cavity
S01.521	Laceration with foreign body of lip
S01.522	Laceration with foreign body of oral cavity
S01.541	Puncture wound with foreign body of lip
S01.542	Puncture wound with foreign body of oral cavity

14. Oral Neoplasms

Malignant: Lip

C00.0	Malignant neoplasm of external upper lip
C00.1	Malignant neoplasm of external lower lip
C00.2	Malignant neoplasm of external lip, unspecified
C00.3	Malignant neoplasm of upper lip, inner aspect
C00.4	Malignant neoplasm of lower lip, inner aspect
C00.5	Malignant neoplasm of lip, unspecified, inner aspect
C00.6	Malignant neoplasm of commissure of lip, unspecified
C00.8	Malignant neoplasm of overlapping sites of lip
C00.9	Malignant neoplasm of lip, unspecified

C44.01	Basal cell carcinoma of skin of lip
C44.02	Squamous cell carcinoma of skin of lip
C44.09	Other specified malignant neoplasm of skin of lip

Malignant: Tongue

C01	Malignant neoplasm of base of tongue
C02.0	Malignant neoplasm of dorsal surface of tongue
C02.1	Malignant neoplasm of border of tongue
C02.2	Malignant neoplasm of ventral surface of tongue
C02.3	Malignant neoplasm of anterior two-thirds of tongue, part unspecified
C02.8	Malignant neoplasm of overlapping sites of tongue

Malignant: Gums

C03.0	Malignant neoplasm of upper gum
C03.1	Malignant neoplasm of lower gum
C03.9	Malignant neoplasm of gum, unspecified

Malignant: Floor of the Mouth

C04.0	Malignant neoplasm of anterior floor of mouth
C04.1	Malignant neoplasm of lateral floor of mouth
C04.8	Malignant neoplasm of overlapping sites of floor of mouth
C04.9	Malignant neoplasm of floor of mouth, unspecified

Malignant: Palate

C05.0	Malignant neoplasm of hard palate
C05.1	Malignant neoplasm of soft palate
C05.8	Malignant neoplasm of overlapping sites of palate
C05.9	Malignant neoplasm of palate, unspecified

Malignant: Oropharyngeal Region

C05.2	Malignant neoplasm of uvula
C02.4	Malignant neoplasm of lingual tonsil
C09.0	Malignant neoplasm of tonsillar fossa
C09.1	Malignant neoplasm of tonsillar pillar (anterior) (posterior)
C09.8	Malignant neoplasm of overlapping sites of tonsil

C09.9	Malignant neoplasm of tonsil, unspecified
C10.0	Malignant neoplasm of vallecula
C10.1	Malignant neoplasm of anterior surface of epiglottis
C10.2	Malignant neoplasm of lateral wall of oropharynx
C10.3	Malignant neoplasm of posterior wall of oropharynx
C10.4	Malignant neoplasm of branchial cleft
C10.8	Malignant neoplasm of overlapping sites of oropharynx
C10.9	Malignant neoplasm of oropharynx, unspecified

Malignant: Other Areas

C06.0	Malignant neoplasm of cheek mucosa
C06.1	Malignant neoplasm of vestibule of mouth
C06.2	Malignant neoplasm of retromolar area
C06.80	Malignant neoplasm of overlapping sites of unspecified parts of mouth
C06.89	Malignant neoplasm of overlapping sites of other parts of mouth
C06.9	Malignant neoplasm of mouth, unspecified
C41.0	Malignant neoplasm of bones of skull and face
C41.1	Malignant neoplasm of mandible
C76.0	Malignant neoplasm of head, face and neck

Malignant: Salivary Glands

C07	Malignant neoplasm of parotid gland
C08.0	Malignant neoplasm of submandibular gland
C08.1	Malignant neoplasm of sublingual gland
C08.9	Malignant neoplasm of major salivary gland, unspecified

Carcinoma in Situ

D00.00	Carcinoma in situ of oral cavity, unspecified site
D00.01	Carcinoma in situ of labial mucosa and vermilion border
D00.02	Carcinoma in situ of buccal mucosa
D00.03	Carcinoma in situ of gingiva and edentulous alveolar ridge
D00.04	Carcinoma in situ of soft palate
D00.05	Carcinoma in situ of hard palate
D00.06	Carcinoma in situ of floor of mouth

D00.07	Carcinoma in situ of tongue
D00.08	Carcinoma in situ of pharynx
D04.0	Carcinoma in situ of skin of lip

Benign Neoplasms

D10.0	Benign neoplasm of lip
D10.1	Benign neoplasm of tongue
D10.2	Benign neoplasm of floor of mouth
D10.30	Benign neoplasm of unspecified part of mouth
D10.39	Benign neoplasm of other parts of mouth
D10.4	Benign neoplasm of tonsil
D10.5	Benign neoplasm of other parts of oropharynx

15. Pathologies

Jaw Related

M27.0	Developmental disorders of jaws
M27.1	Giant cell granuloma, central
M27.2	Inflammatory conditions of jaws
M27.3	Alveolitis of jaws
M27.40	Unspecified cyst of jaw
M27.49	Other cysts of jaw
M27.8	Other specified diseases of jaws

Cysts

K09.0	Developmental odontogenic cysts
K09.1	Developmental (nonodontogenic) cysts of oral region
K09.8	Other cysts of oral region, not elsewhere classified

Salivary Glands

K11.0	Atrophy of salivary gland
K11.1	Hypertrophy of salivary gland
K11.21	Acute sialoadenitis
K11.22	Acute recurrent sialoadenitis
K11.23	Chronic sialoadenitis
K11.3	Abscess of salivary gland

K11.4	Fistula of salivary gland
K11.5	Sialolithiasis
K11.6	Mucocele of salivary gland
K11.7	Disturbances of salivary secretion
K11.8	Other diseases of salivary glands

Lips and Oral Mucosa

K13.1	Cheek and lip biting
K13.21	Leukoplakia of oral mucosa, including tongue
K13.22	Minimal keratinized residual ridge mucosa
K13.23	Excessive keratinized residual ridge mucosa
K13.24	Leukokeratosis nicotina palate
K13.29	Other disturbances of oral epithelium, including tongue
K13.3	Hairy leukoplakia
K13.4	Granuloma and granuloma-like lesions of oral mucosa
K13.5	Oral submucous fibrosis
K13.6	Irritative hyperplasia of oral mucosa
K13.79	Other lesions of oral mucosa

Tongue

K14.0	Glossitis
K14.1	Geographic tongue
K14.2	Median rhomboid glossitis
K14.3	Hypertrophy of tongue papillae
K14.4	Atrophy of tongue papillae
K14.5	Plicated tongue
K14.6	Glossodynia
K14.8	Other diseases of tongue

Skin and Subcutaneous Tissues

L40.52	Psoriatric arthritis mutilans
L40.54	Psoriatic juvenile arthropathy
L40.59	Other psoriatic arthropathy
L43.9	Lichen planus, unspecified
L90.5	Scar conditions and fibrosis of skin

Musculoskeletal System and Connective Tissue

M06.9	Rheumatoid arthritis, unspecified
M08.00	Unspecified juvenile rheumatoid arthritis of unspecified site
M24.20	Disorder of ligament, unspecified site
M32.10	Systemic lupus erythematosus, organ or system involvement unspecified
M35.00	Sicca syndrome [Sjögren], unspecified
M35.7	Hypermobility syndrome
M43.6	Torticollis
M45.9	Ankylosing spondylitis of unspecified sites in spine
M54.2	Cervicalgia
M60.9	Myositis, unspecified
M62.40	Contracture of muscle, unspecified site
M62.81	Muscle weakness (generalized)
M62.838	Other muscle spasm
M65.9	Synovitis and tenosynovitis, unspecified
S00.511A	Abrasion of lip, initial encounter
S00.511D	Abrasion of lip, subsequent encounter
S00.511S	Abrasion of lip, sequela
M79.2	Neuralgia and neuritis, unspecified
M87.00	Idiopathic aseptic necrosis of unspecified bone
M87.180	Osteonecrosis due to drugs, jaw

16. Medical Findings Related to Dental Treatment

Communicable Diseases

A69.20	Lyme disease, unspecified
B00.0	Eczema herpeticum (Kaposi's varicelliform eruption)
B00.1	Herpesviral vesicular dermatitis
B00.2	Herpesviral gingivostomatitis and pharyngotonsillitis
B37.0	Candidal stomatitis (Oral Thrush)

Diabetes

E08.630   Diabetes mellitus due to underlying condition with periodontal disease

E08.638   Diabetes mellitus due to underlying condition with other oral complications

E09.630   Drug or chemical induced diabetes mellitus with periodontal disease

E09.638   Drug or chemical induced diabetes mellitus with other oral complications

E10.630   Type 1 diabetes mellitus with periodontal disease

E10.638   Type 1 diabetes mellitus with other oral complications

E10.9   Type 1 diabetes mellitus without complications

E11.630   Type 2 diabetes mellitus with periodontal disease

E11.638   Type 2 diabetes mellitus with other oral complications

E11.9   Type 2 diabetes mellitus without complications

E13.630   Other specified diabetes mellitus with periodontal disease

E13.638   Other specified diabetes mellitus with other oral complications

R73.01   Impaired fasting glucose

R73.02   Impaired glucose tolerance (oral)

R73.03   Prediabetes

R73.09   Other abnormal glucose

R73.9   Hyperglycemia, unspecified

Substance Abuse/Tobacco Use

Z71.6   Tobacco abuse counseling

Z72.0   Tobacco use

F17.200   Nicotine dependence, unspecified, uncomplicated

F17.210   Nicotine dependence, cigarettes, uncomplicated

F17.220   Nicotine dependence, chewing tobacco, uncomplicated

F17.290   Nicotine dependence, other tobacco products, uncomplicated

New Diseases of Uncertain Etiology

U07.0   Vaping related disorder

Substance Abuse/Alcohol Use

F10.10	Alcohol abuse, uncomplicated
F10.11	Alcohol abuse, in remission
F10.129	Alcohol abuse with intoxication, unspecified
F10.19	Alcohol abuse with unspecified alcohol-induced disorder

Family History

Z80.0	Family history of malignant neoplasm of digestive organs
Z81.0	Family history of intellectual disabilities
Z81.1	Family history of alcohol abuse and dependence
Z81.2	Family history of tobacco abuse and dependence
Z81.3	Family history of other psychoactive substance abuse and dependence
Z81.4	Family history of other substance abuse and dependence
Z81.8	Family history of other mental and behavioral disorders
Z83.0	Family history of human immunodeficiency virus [HIV] disease
Z83.2	Family history of diseases of the blood and blood-forming organs and certain disorders involving the immune mechanism
Z83.3	Family history of diabetes mellitus
Z83.49	Family history of other endocrine, nutritional and metabolic diseases
Z83.79	Family history of other diseases of the digestive system

Personal History

F41.9	Anxiety disorder, unspecified
R45.0	Nervousness
P92.9	Feeding problem of newborn, unspecified
Z85.00	Personal history of malignant neoplasm of unspecified digestive organ
Z85.810	Personal history of malignant neoplasm of tongue
Z85.818	Personal history of malignant neoplasm of other sites of lip, oral cavity, and pharynx
Z85.819	Personal history of malignant neoplasm of unspecified site of lip, oral cavity, and pharynx
Z85.830	Personal history of malignant neoplasm of bone
Z85.831	Personal history of malignant neoplasm of soft tissue

Z86.003	Personal history of in-situ neoplasm of oral cavity, esophagus and stomach.
Z87.730	Personal history (corrected) of cleft lip and palate
Z87.738	Personal history of other specified (corrected) congenital malformations of digestive system
Z88.0	Allergy status to penicillin
Z88.1	Allergy status to other antibiotic agents status
Z88.2	Allergy status to sulfonamides status
Z88.3	Allergy status to other anti-infective agents status
Z88.4	Allergy status to anesthetic agent status
Z88.5	Allergy status to narcotic agent status
Z88.6	Allergy status to analgesic agent status
Z88.7	Allergy status to serum and vaccine status
Z88.8	Allergy status to other drugs, medicaments and biological substances status
Z88.9	Allergy status to unspecified drugs, medicaments and biological substances status
Z91.09	Other allergy status, other than to drugs and biological substances
Z91.19	Patient's noncompliance with other medical treatment and regimen
Z91.89	Other specified personal risk factors, not elsewhere classified
Z92.3	Personal history of irradiation (therapeutic radiation)
Z92.83	Personal history of failed moderate sedation (concious sedation)
Z92.84	Personal history of unintended awareness under general anesthesia
Z92.89	Personal history of other medical treatment

Nerve Disorders

G50.0	Trigeminal neuralgia
G50.1	Atypical face pain
G50.8	Other disorders of trigeminal nerve
G51.8	Other disorders of facial nerve
G52.1	Disorders of glossopharyngeal nerve
G52.3	Disorder of hypoglossal nerve
G52.8	Disorder of other specified cranial nerve

Sinusitis	
J32.0	Chronic maxillary sinusitis
J32.1	Chronic frontal sinusitis
J32.9	Chronic sinusitis, unspecified
R68.2	Dry mouth, unspecified (Not due to Sicca [Sjögren] syndrome)

Other Specified Health Status	
Z78.1	Physical restraint status
Z78.9	Other specified health status
Z79.01	Long term (current) use of anticoagulants
Z79.02	Long term (current) use of antithrombotics/antiplatelets
Z79.1	Long term (current) use of non-steroidal anti-inflammatories (NSAID)
Z79.2	Long term (current) use of antibiotics
Z79.4	Long term (current) use of insulin
Z79.51	Long term (current) use of inhaled steroids
Z79.52	Long term (current) use of systemic steroids
Z79.82	Long term (current) use of aspirin
Z79.83	Long term (current) use of bisphosphonates
Z79.84	Long term (current) use of oral hypoglycemic drugs
Z79.891	Long term (current) use of opiate analgesic
Z79.899	Other long term (current) drug therapy

17. Social Determinants

Problems Related to Education and Literacy	
Z55.0	Illiteracy and low-level literacy
Z55.1	Schooling unavailable and unattainable
Z55.3	Underachievement in school
Z55.4	Educational maladjustment and discord with teachers and classmates
Z55.8	Other problems related to education and literacy
Z55.9	Problems related to education and literacy, unspecified

Problems Related to Housing and Economic Circumstances

Z59.0	Homelessness
Z59.1	Inadequate housing
Z59.4	Lack of adequate food and safe drinking water
Z59.5	Extreme poverty
Z59.6	Low income
Z59.7	Insufficient social insurance and welfare support
Z59.8	Other problems related to housing and economic circumstances

Problems Related to Social Environment

Z60.0	Problems of adjustment to life-cycle transitions
Z60.2	Problems related to living alone
Z60.8	Other problems related to social environment

18. Symptoms and Disorders Pertinent to Orthodontia Cases

Pain

G24.3	Spasmodic toticcollis
G24.4	Idiopathic orofacial dystonia (Orofacial dyskinesia)
G44.1	Vascular headache, not elsewhere classified
G44.201	Tension-type headache, unspecified, intractable
G44.209	Tension-type headache, unspecified, not intractable
G44.211	Episodic tension-type headache, intractable
G44.219	Episodic tension-type headache, not intractable
G44.221	Chronic tension-type headache, intractable
G44.229	Chronic tension-type headache, not intractable
H57.11	Ocular pain, right eye
H57.12	Ocular pain, left eye
H57.13	Ocular pain, bilateral
M79.11	Myalgia of mastication muscle
M79.12	Myalgia of auxiliary muscles, head and neck
M79.18	Myalgia, other site

Migraine

G43.001	Migraine without aura, not intractable, with status migrainosus
G43.009	Migraine without aura, not intractable, without status migrainosus
G43.011	Migraine without aura, intractable, with status migrainosus
G43.019	Migraine without aura, intractable, without status migrainosus
G43.101	Migraine with aura, not intractable, with status migrainosus
G43.109	Migraine with aura, not intractable, without status migrainosus
G43.111	Migraine with aura, not-intractable, with status migrainosus
G43.119	Migraine with aura, intractable, without status migrainosus
G43.701	Chronic migraine without aura, not-intractable, with status migrainosus
G43.719	Chronic migraine without aura, not-intractable, without status migrainosus
G43.801	Other migraine, not intractable, with status migrainosus
G43.809	Other migraine, not intractable, without status migrainosus
G43.811	Other migraine, intractable, with status migrainosus
G43.819	Other migraine, intractable, without status migrainosus
G44.1	Vascular headache, not elsewhere classified

Ears and Larynx

H92.01	Otalgia, right ear
H92.02	Otalgia, left ear
H92.03	Otalgia, bilateral
H93.11	Tinnitus, right ear
H93.12	Tinnitus, left ear
H93.13	Tinnitus, bilateral
J38.5	Laryngeal spasm

Craniofacial

Q67.0	Congenital facial asymmetry
Q67.4	Other congenital deformities of skull, face and jaw
Q74.0	Other congenital malformations of upper limb(s), including shoulder girdle (Includes Cleidocranial dysostosis)

Q75.0	Craniosynostosis (aka Pierrre Robin Sequence)
Q75.1	Craniofacial dysostosis (Crouzon's disease [syndrome])
Q75.2	Hypertelorism
Q75.3	Macrocephaply
Q75.4	Mandibulofacial dysostosis (Treacher Collins syndrome)
Q75.5	Oculomandibular dysostosis
Q75.8	Other specified malformations of skull and face bones
Q75.9	Congenital malformation of skull and face bones, unspecified
Q87.0	Congenital malformation syndromes predominantly affecting facial appearance (Includes – Acrocephalopolysyndactyly [aka Apert Syndrome and Pfeiffer Syndrome])
Q87.19	Other congenital malformation syndromes predominantly associated with short stature (Includes – Noonan syndrome)

Turners Syndrome

Q96.0	Karyotype 45, X
Q96.2	Karyotype 46, X with abnormal sex chromosome, except iso (Xq)
Q96.3	Mosaicism, 45, X/46, XX or XY
Q96.4	Mosaicism, 45, X/other cell line(s) with abnormal sex chromosome
Q96.8	Other variants of Turner's Sydrome
Q96.9	Turner's Syndrome, unspecified

Other

E22.0	Acromegaly and pituitary gigantism
E23.0	Hypopituitarism (Includes – Isolated deficiency of growth hormone)
G25.3	Myoclonus
R42.	Dizziness and giddiness (Includes – Light-headedness)
K00.9	Disorder of tooth development (and eruption), unspecified (aka Disorder of odontogenesis NOS)

Section 4

Alphabetic Index to the CDT Code

Term	Code(s)	Page(s)
A		
A1c testing	D0411	8
Abscess, incision and drainage, all types	D7510, D7511, D7520, D7521	65
Abutments	Also see **Retainers**	
for implants	D6051, D6056, D6057	49
Accession of tissue	D0472–D0474	10
Acid etch; part of resin procedure	No separate code	
Adhesives, bonding agents (resin and and amalgam bonding agents); part of restorative procedure	No separate code	
Adjunctive General Services (Category of Service)	D9000–D9999	77–84
Adjunctive pre-diagnostic test	D0431	9
Adjust		
prosthetic appliance	D5992	39
orthodontic retainer	D8681	75
Allograft, soft tissue	D4275, D7955	31, 71
Alveoloplasty	D7310, D7311, D7320, D7321	63
Alveolus, fracture	D7670, D7671, D7770, D7771	66, 67
Amalgam restorations	D2140–D2161	16

Term	Code(s)	Page(s)
Amalgam and resin bonding agents (part of restorative procedure)	No separate code	
Analgesia		
inhalation of nitrous oxide	D9230	78
non-intravenous conscious sedation	D9248	78
Anchorage device, temporary		
requiring flap	D7293	62
without flap	D7294	62
screw retained plate requiring flap	D7292	62
Anesthesia		
evaluation for...general	D9219	77
general	D9222, D9223	78
local	D9210, D9215	77
regional	D9211	77
trigeminal division block	D9212	77
Ankyloglossia	See **frenectomy/frenotomy (frenulectomy)**	
Apexification/recalcification	D3351–D3353	23
Apexogenesis	D3222	21
Apically positioned flap	D4245	29
Apicoectomy	D3410–D3473	24
Appliance removal (not by dentist who placed)	D7997	72
Arthrocentesis	D7870	68
Appointment		
cancelled	D9987	82
missed	D9986	82
Arthroplasty	D7865	68
Arthroscopy	D7872–D7877	68
Arthrotomy	D7860	68
Assessment of a patient	D0191	5
Athletic mouthguard	D9941	81
Autologous blood concentrate (collection and application)	D7921	69

4 | Alphabetic Index to the CDT Code

Term	Code(s)	Page(s)
Carrier		
fluoride gel	D5986	46
periodontal medicament	D5995–D5996	47
radiation	D5983	47
vesiculobolus medicament	D5991	47
Case presentation	D9450	79
Cast post and core	D2952	20
each additional (same tooth)	D2953	20
Casts, diagnostic (study models)	D0470	9
Cephalometric image	D0340; D0702	6, 7
Changes in structure – enamel/dentin/ cementum	D0600	9
Cleaning and inspection of a removable appliance	D9932–D9935	81
Clot stabilization (hemostasis)	D7922	69
Collection and application of autologous blood concentrate	D7921	69
Combined connective tissue and double pedicle graft	D4276	31
Complications, post-surgical	D9930	81
Composite resin	**See Resin-based composite** (direct and indirect)	
Comprehensive orthodontics	D8070–D8090	74
Condylectomy	D7840	67
Cone Beam – CT		
image capture and interpretation	D0364–D0368	6
image capture only	D0380–D0384	7
interpretation and report only	D0391	8
post processing image or image sets	D0393–D0395	8
Connector bar		
dental implant supported	D6055	49
fixed partial denture	D6920	59
Conscious sedation	D9239, D9243, D9248	78

Term	Code(s)	Page(s)
Dressing change, periodontal, unscheduled	D4920	33
Drugs		
therapeutic parenteral, single administration	D9610	80
therapeutic parental, two or more administrations	D9612	80
infiltration of sustained release therapeutic drug, single or multiple sites	D9613	80
drugs or medicaments	D9630	80
Dry socket/localized osteitis	D9930	81

E

Term	Code(s)	Page(s)
Emergency treatment	D0140, D9110	3, 77
Enamel microabrasion	D9970	82
Enameloplasty	D9971	82
Endodontics (Category of Service)	D3000–D3999	21–26
Endodontic endosseous implant	D3460	25
Equilibration (occlusal adjustment)	D9951, D9952	82
Eruption of teeth		
mobilization, surgical	D7282	61
placement of device to aid eruption	D7283	61
Evaluations		
periodic – established patient	D0120	3
limited – problem focused	D0140	3
for patient under 3 years & counseling with primary caregiver	D0145	3
comprehensive – new or established patient	D0150	3
detailed and extensive – problem focused, by report	D0160	4
re-evaluation – limited	D0170	4
re-evaluation – post-operative office visit	D0171	4

Term	Code(s)	Page(s)
maxilla – open (compound) fractures		
open reduction	D7710	66
closed reduction	D7720	66
maxilla – closed (simple) fractures		
open reduction	D7610	66
closed reduction	D7620	66
Frenectomy/frenotomy (frenulectomy)	D7961–D7962	71
buccal/labial	D7961	71
lingual	D7962	71
Frenuloplasty	D7963	71
Full mouth series	D0210; D0709	5, 7

G

Term	Code(s)	Page(s)
Genetic testing		
sample collection	D0422	9
specimen analysis	D0423	9
Gingiva, pericoronal, removal of	D7971	71
Gingival flap	D4240, D4241	28
Gingival Irrigation	D4921	33
Gingivectomy/gingivoplasty	D4210–D4212	27
Glass ionomers (resin restorations)	D2330–D2394	16
Glucose meter – blood level test	D0412	8
Gold foil	D2410–D2430	17
Graft		
bone replacement	D4263, D4264, D6103, D6104, D7953	29, 30, 49, 70
combined connective tissue and double pedicle	D4276	31
free soft tissue	D4277–D4278	32
maxillofacial soft/hard tissue	D7955	71
osseous, osteoperiosteal, or cartilage	D7950	70
pedicle soft tissue	D4270	31
periradicular	D3428, D3429	25

Term	Code(s)	Page(s)
Internal root repair	D3333	22
Interpretation of diagnostic image (different practitioner)	D0391	8
Intravenous moderate (conscious) sedation/analgesia	D9239, D9243	78
Irrigation (gingival)	D4921	33

J

Joint reconstruction	D7858	67

K

No "K" terms

L

Term	Code(s)	Page(s)
Labial veneer	D2960–D2962	20
Laser	No separate code – part of dental procedure code that appropriately describes the service provided	
Lateral exostosis	D7471	65
LeFort I	D7946, D7947	69, 70
LeFort II; LeFort III	D7948, D7949	70
Lesions, surgical excision		
intra-osseous lesions	D7440–D7461	64
soft tissue	D7410–D7415, D7465	64
Limited orthodontic treatment	D8010–D8040	73
Localized osteitis/dry socket	D9930	81

M

Term	Code(s)	Page(s)
Maintenance and cleaning of prosthesis	D5993	39
Malar bone, repair of fracture	D7650, D7660, D7750, D7760	66
Malocclusion, correction of	D8000–D8999	73–76
Mandible, fracture of	D7630–D7640, D7730–D7740	66

4 | Alphabetic Index to the CDT Code

Term	Code(s)	Page(s)
Non-intravenous moderate (conscious) sedation	D9248	78
Non-odontogenic cyst	D7460, D7461	64
Nursing home, (house/extended care facility visit)	D9410	79
Nutritional counseling	D1310	12

O

Term	Code(s)	Page(s)
Obturator		
post-surgical	D5932	42
refitting	D5933	42
surgical	D5931	43
Occlusal adjustment (equilibration)	D9951, D9952	82
Occlusal image, intraoral	D0240	5
Occlusal guard		
hard appliance, full arch	D9944	81
soft appliance, full arch	D9945	81
hard appliance, partial arch	D9946	81
adjustment	D9943	81
reline or repair	D9942	81
Occlusal orthotic device	D7880	68
Occlusal orthotic device adjustment	D7881	68
Occlusion analysis	D9950	81
Odontogenic cyst	D7450, D7451	64
Odontoplasty (enameloplasty)	D9971	82
Office visit	D9430, D9440	79
Onlay		
fixed partial denture retainers	D6610–D6615, D6634	57
metallic	D2542–D2544	17
porcelain/ceramic	D2642–D2644	17
resin-based composite	D2662–D2664	18
Operculectomy	D7971	71

4 | Alphabetic Index to the CDT Code

Term	Code(s)	Page(s)

P

Term	Code(s)	Page(s)
Palliative treatment	D9110	77
Panoramic image	D0330; D0701	6, 7
Partial dentures, fixed	See **fixed partial denture**	
Partial dentures, removable		
adjustments	D5421, D5422	35
cast metal framework, resin base	D5213, D5214	34
flexible base	D5225, D5226	35
interim	D5820, D5821	37
overdenture	D5863–D5866	38
reline	D5740, D5741, D5760, D5761	37
repair	D5611, D5612, D5621, D5622–D5671	36
resin base	D5211, D5212	34
unilateral	D5282–D5286	35
Patient		
Screening	D0190	5
Assessment	D0191	5
Patient record duplication/copying	D9961	82
Perforation defect, internal repair	D3333	22
Periapical images	D0220–D0230; D0707	5, 7
Pericoronal gingival excision	D7971	71
Periodic orthodontic treatment visit	D8670	75
Periodontal evaluation	D0180	4
Periodontal maintenance	D4910	33
Periodontal medicament carrier	D5995, D5996	47
Periodontics (Category of Service)	D4000–D4999	27–33
Periradicular surgery/apicoectomy	D3410–D3426	24
Pharmacologic agents	See **Drugs**	
Photographic images, diagnostic		
2D (two-dimensional)	D0350; D0702, D0703	6, 7
3D (three-dimensional)	D0351, D0704	6, 7

4 | Alphabetic Index to the CDT Code

Term	Code(s)	Page(s)
maxillofacial (Category of Service)	D5900–D5999	39–47
removable (Category of Service)	D5000–D5899	34–38
Protective restoration	D2940	19
Provisional		
single crown	D2799	18
pontic (FPD)	D6253	56
implant crown	D6085	55
retainer crown (FPD)	D6793	58
Pulp cap	D3110, D3120	21
Pulp vitality tests	D0460	9
Pulpal debridement	D3221	21
Pupal regeneration	D3355–D3357	23
Pulpal therapy, primary teeth	D3230, D3240	22
Pulpotomy		
therapeutic (excluding final restoration)	D3220	21
partial for apexogenesis	D3222	21

Q

No "Q" terms.

R

Radiation		
carrier	D5983	47
cone locator	D5985	44
shield	D5984	45
Radiographic/surgical implant index	D6190	48
Radiographs		
image capture and interpretation	D0210–D0340	5–6
interpretation and report only	D0391	8
Reattach tooth fragment	D2921	19
Recalcification/apexification	D3351–D3353	23
Re-cement		
bridge	D6930	59

S

Term	Code(s)	Page(s)

T

Teledentistry

Synchronous; real time encounter	D9995	83
Asynchronous ("store and forward")	D9996	84

Temporomandibular joint (TMJ)

manipulation	D7830	67
radiographs	D0320, D0321	6
reduction	D7810, D7820	67
surgical discectomy	D7850	67
treatment	D7810–D7899	67–68

Temporomandibular joint dysfunction – non-invasive physical therapies	D9130	77
Thumb sucking appliance	D8210, D8220	75
Tissue conditioning	D5850, D5851	37
Tissue, excision of hyperplastic	D7970	71

Titanium

crown, FPD retainer	D6794	58
crown, single unit	D2794	18
implant abutment supported	D6094, D6097	51
implant abutment supported for FPD	D6194	53
implant supported	D6065, D6088	52
implant supported for FPD	D6067, D6099	52, 54
inlay, FPD retainer	D6624	57
onlay, FPD retainer	D6634	57
pontic	D6214	56

Tobacco counseling	D1320	12
Tomographic survey	D0322	6
Tongue thrusting appliance	D8210, D8220	75

Tooth, natural

caries susceptibility test	D0425	9
extraction	D7111, D7140, D7210–D7250	60–61

Term	Code(s)	Page(s)

W

Wax-up (diagnostic)	D9950	81
Wedge – mesial/distal	D4274	31
Whitening	See **Bleaching**	
Wounds, treatment of	D7910–D7912	69

X

X-rays	See **Diagnostic Imaging**	

Y

No "Y" terms.

Z

Zirconia / Zirconium	Use applicable "porcelain/ceramic" prosthesis code from Restorative, Prosthodontic or Implant categories	
Zygomatic arch		
simple fracture treatment		
open reduction	D7650	66
closed reduction	D7660	66
compound fracture treatment		
open reduction	D7750	66
closed reduction	D7760	66
Zygomatic implant	D7994	72

Section 5
Numeric Index to the CDT Code

CDT Category		Code Entry Change (when applicable)		CDT Category		Code Entry Change (when applicable)	
Code	Page	Addition Revision Deletion Editorial	Page	Code	Page	Addition Revision Deletion Editorial	Page
I. Diagnostic				D0322	6		
D0120	3	Editorial	88	D0330	6		
D0140	3			D0340	6		
D0145	3			D0350	6		
D0150	3	Editorial	88	D0351	6		
D0160	4			D0364	6		
D0170	4			D0365	6		
D0171	4			D0366	6		
D0180	4			D0367	6		
D0190	5			D0368	6		
D0191	5			D0369	6		
D0210	5			D0370	6		
D0220	5			D0371	6		
D0230	5			D0380	7		
D0240	5			D0381	7		
D0250	5			D0382	7		
D0251	5			D0383	7		
D0270	5			D0384	7		
D0272	5			D0385	7		
D0273	5			D0386	7		
D0274	6			D0391	8		
D0277	6			D0393	8		
D0310	6			D0394	8		
D0320	6			D0395	8		
D0321	6			D0411	8		

CDT Category		Code Entry Change (when applicable)		CDT Category		Code Entry Change (when applicable)	
Code	Page	Addition Revision Deletion Editorial	Page	Code	Page	Addition Revision Deletion Editorial	Page
D0412	8			D0702	7	Addition	87
D0414	8			D0703	7	Addition	87
D0415	8			D0704	7	Addition	87
D0416	8			D0705	7	Addition	87
D0417	8			D0706	7	Addition	87
D0418	8			D0707	7	Addition	87
D0419	8			D0708	7	Addition	87
D0422	9			D0709	7	Addition	87
D0423	9			D0999	11		
D0425	9			II. Preventive			
D0431	9			D1110	12	Revision	89
D0460	9			D1120	12	Revision	89
D0470	9			D1206	12		
D0472	10			D1208	12		
D0473	10			D1310	12		
D0474	10			D1320	12		
D0475	10			D1321	12	Addition	89
D0476	10			D1330	13		
D0477	10			D1351	13		
D0478	11			D1352	13		
D0479	11			D1353	13		
D0480	10			D1354	13		
D0481	11			D1355	13	Addition	89
D0482	11			D1510	13		
D0483	11			D1516	13		
D0484	11			D1517	13		
D0485	11			D1520	13		
D0486	10			D1526	13		
D0502	11			D1527	13		
D0600	9			D1551	13		
D0601	9			D1552	13		
D0602	9			D1553	14		
D0603	9			D1556	14		
D0604	9	Addition	87	D1557	14	Revision	89
D0605	9	Addition	87	D1558	14	Revision	89
D0701	7	Addition	87	D1575	14		

CDT Category		Code Entry Change (when applicable)		CDT Category		Code Entry Change (when applicable)	
Code	Page	Addition Revision Deletion Editorial	Page	Code	Page	Addition Revision Deletion Editorial	Page
D1999	14			D2710	18		
III. Restorative				D2712	18		
D2140	16			D2720	18		
D2150	16			D2721	18		
D2160	16			D2722	18		
D2161	16			D2740	18		
D2330	16			D2750	18		
D2331	16			D2751	18		
D2332	16			D2752	18		
D2335	16			D2753	18		
D2390	16			D2780	18		
D2391	16			D2781	18		
D2392	16			D2782	18		
D2393	16			D2783	18		
D2394	16			D2790	18		
D2410	17			D2791	18		
D2420	17			D2792	18		
D2430	17			D2794	18		
D2510	17			D2799	18		
D2520	17			D2910	19		
D2530	17			D2915	19		
D2542	17			D2920	19		
D2543	17			D2921	19		
D2544	17			D2928	19	Addition	90
D2610	17			D2929	19		
D2620	17			D2930	19		
D2630	17			D2931	19		
D2642	17			D2932	19		
D2643	17			D2933	19		
D2644	17			D2934	19		
D2650	17			D2940	19		
D2651	17			D2941	19		
D2652	17			D2949	19		
D2662	18			D2950	19		
D2663	18			D2951	20		
D2664	18			D2952	20		

CDT Category		Code Entry Change (when applicable)		CDT Category		Code Entry Change (when applicable)	
Code	Page	Addition Revision Deletion Editorial	Page	Code	Page	Addition Revision Deletion Editorial	Page
D2953	20			D3356	23		
D2954	20			D3357	23		
D2955	20			D3410	24		
D2957	20			D3421	24		
D2960	20	Editorial	90	D3425	24		
D2961	20	Editorial	90	D3426	24		
D2962	20	Editorial	90	D3427		Deletion	
D2971	20			D3428	25		
D2975	20			D3429	25		
D2980	20			D3430	25		
D2981	20			D3431	25		
D2982	20			D3432	25		
D2983	20			D3450	25		
D2990	19			D3460	25		
D2999	20			D3470	25		
IV. Endodontics				D3471	24	Addition	91
D3110	21			D3472	24	Addition	91
D3120	21			D3473	24	Addition	91
D3220	21			D3501	24	Addition	91
D3221	21			D3502	25	Addition	91
D3222	21			D3503	25	Addition	91
D3230	22			D3910	26		
D3240	22			D3920	26		
D3310	22			D3950	26		
D3320	22			D3999	26		
D3330	22			V. Periodontics			
D3331	22			D4210	27		
D3332	22			D4211	27		
D3333	22			D4212	27		
D3346	23			D4230	28		
D3347	23			D4231	28		
D3348	23			D4240	28		
D3351	23			D4241	28		
D3352	23			D4245	29		
D3353	23			D4249	29		
D3355	23			D4260	29		

CDT Category		Code Entry Change (when applicable)		CDT Category		Code Entry Change (when applicable)	
Code	Page	Addition Revision Deletion Editorial	Page	Code	Page	Addition Revision Deletion Editorial	Page
D4261	29			D5221	34		
D4263	29			D5222	34		
D4264	30			D5223	35		
D4265	30			D5224	35		
D4266	30			D5225	35	Editorial	93
D4267	30			D5226	35	Editorial	93
D4268	30			D5282	35	Editorial	93
D4270	31			D5283	35	Editorial	93
D4273	31			D5284	35	Editorial	93
D4274	31			D5286	35	Editorial	93
D4275	31			D5410	35		
D4276	31			D5411	35		
D4277	32			D5421	35		
D4278	32			D5422	35		
D4283	31			D5511	36		
D4285	31			D5512	36		
D4320	32			D5520	36		
D4321	32			D5611	36		
D4341	32			D5612	36		
D4342	32			D5621	36		
D4346	33			D5622	36		
D4355	33			D5630	36		
D4381	33			D5640	36		
D4910	33			D5650	36		
D4920	33			D5660	36		
D4921	33			D5670	36		
D4999	33			D5671	36		
VI. Prosthodontics (removable)				D5710	36		
D5110	34			D5711	36		
D5120	34			D5720	36		
D5130	34			D5721	36		
D5140	34			D5730	37	Editorial	93
D5211	34			D5731	37	Editorial	93
D5212	34			D5740	37	Editorial	93
D5213	34			D5741	37	Editorial	94
D5214	34			D5750	37	Editorial	94

CDT Category		Code Entry Change (when applicable)		CDT Category		Code Entry Change (when applicable)	
Code	Page	Addition Revision Deletion Editorial	Page	Code	Page	Addition Revision Deletion Editorial	Page
D5751	37	Editorial	94	D5933	42		
D5760	37	Editorial	94	D5934	41		
D5761	37	Editorial	94	D5935	41		
D5810	37			D5936	42		
D5811	37			D5937	46		
D5820	37	Editorial	94	D5951	40		
D5821	37	Editorial	94	D5952	45		
D5850	37			D5953	45		
D5851	37			D5954	44		
D5862	37			D5955	44		
D5863	38			D5958	44		
D5864	38			D5959	44		
D5865	38			D5960	45		
D5866	38			D5982	46		
D5867	38			D5983	47		
D5875	38			D5984	45		
D5876	38			D5985	44		
D5899	38			D5986	46		
VII. Maxillofacial Prosthetics				D5987	39		
D5911	40			D5988	46		
D5912	40			D5991	47		
D5913	41			D5992	39		
D5914	39			D5993	39		
D5915	43			D5994		Deletion	
D5916	43			D5995	47	Addition	95
D5919	40			D5996	47	Addition	95
D5922	42			D5999	47		
D5923	43			VIII. Implant Services			
D5924	39			D6010	48		
D5925	39			D6011	48	Revision	96
D5926	41			D6012	48		
D5927	39			D6013	48		
D5928	44			D6040	48		
D5929	40			D6050	49		
D5931	43			D6051	49		
D5932	42			D6052		Deletion	

CDT Category		Code Entry Change (when applicable)		CDT Category		Code Entry Change (when applicable)	
Code	Page	Addition Revision Deletion Editorial	Page	Code	Page	Addition Revision Deletion Editorial	Page
D6055	49			D6094	51		
D6056	49			D6095	55		
D6057	49			D6096	55		
D6058	51			D6097	51		
D6059	51			D6098	54	**Editorial**	96
D6060	51			D6099	54		
D6061	51			D6100	49		
D6062	51			D6101	49		
D6063	51			D6102	49		
D6064	51			D6103	49		
D6065	52			D6104	49		
D6066	52			D6110	50		
D6067	52			D6111	50		
D6068	53			D6112	50		
D6069	53			D6113	50		
D6070	53			D6114	50		
D6071	53			D6115	50		
D6072	53			D6116	50		
D6073	53			D6117	50		
D6074	53			D6118	50		
D6075	54			D6119	50		
D6076	54			D6120	54		
D6077	54			D6121	54		
D6080	55			D6122	54		
D6081	55			D6123	54		
D6082	52			D6190	48		
D6083	52			D6191	50	**Addition**	96
D6084	52			D6192	50	**Addition**	96
D6085	55			D6194	53		
D6086	52			D6195	53		
D6087	52			D6199	55		
D6088	52			IX. Prosthodontics, Fixed			
D6090	55			D6205	56		
D6091	55	**Revision**	96	D6210	56		
D6092	55			D6211	56		
D6093	55			D6212	56		

CDT Category		Code Entry Change (when applicable)		CDT Category		Code Entry Change (when applicable)	
Code	Page	Addition Revision Deletion Editorial	Page	Code	Page	Addition Revision Deletion Editorial	Page
D6214	56			D6750	58		
D6240	56			D6751	58		
D6241	56			D6752	58		
D6242	56			D6753	58		
D6243	56			D6780	58		
D6245	56			D6781	58		
D6250	56			D6782	58		
D6251	56			D6783	58		
D6252	56			D6784	58		
D6253	56			D6790	58		
D6545	57			D6791	58		
D6548	57			D6792	58		
D6549	57			D6793	58		
D6600	57			D6794	58		
D6601	57			D6920	59		
D6602	57			D6930	59		
D6603	57			D6940	59		
D6604	57			D6950	59		
D6605	57			D6980	59		
D6606	57			D6985	59		
D6607	57			D6999	59		
D6608	57			X. Oral & Maxillofacial Surgery			
D6609	57			D7111	60		
D6610	57			D7140	60		
D6611	57			D7210	60		
D6612	57			D7220	60		
D6613	57			D7230	60		
D6614	57			D7240	60		
D6615	57			D7241	60		
D6624	57			D7250	61		
D6634	57			D7251	61		
D6710	58			D7260	61		
D6720	58			D7261	61		
D6721	58			D7270	61		
D6722	58			D7272	61		
D6740	58			D7280	61		

CDT Category		Code Entry Change (when applicable)		CDT Category		Code Entry Change (when applicable)	
Code	Page	Addition Revision Deletion Editorial	Page	Code	Page	Addition Revision Deletion Editorial	Page
D7282	61			D7485	65		
D7283	61			D7490	65		
D7285	62			D7510	65		
D7286	62			D7511	65		
D7287	62			D7520	65		
D7288	62			D7521	65		
D7290	62			D7530	65		
D7291	62			D7540	65		
D7292	62			D7550	65		
D7293	62			D7560	65		
D7294	62			D7610	66		
D7295	62			D7620	66		
D7296	63			D7630	66		
D7297	63			D7640	66		
D7310	63			D7650	66		
D7311	63			D7660	66		
D7320	63			D7670	66		
D7321	63			D7671	66		
D7340	64			D7680	66		
D7350	64			D7710	66		
D7410	64			D7720	66		
D7411	64			D7730	66		
D7412	64			D7740	66		
D7413	64			D7750	66		
D7414	64			D7760	66		
D7415	64			D7770	66		
D7440	64			D7771	66		
D7441	64			D7780	66		
D7450	64			D7810	67		
D7451	64			D7820	67		
D7460	64			D7830	67		
D7461	64			D7840	67		
D7465	64			D7850	67		
D7471	65			D7852	67		
D7472	65			D7854	67		
D7473	65			D7856	67		

CDT Category		Code Entry Change (when applicable)		CDT Category		Code Entry Change (when applicable)	
Code	Page	Addition Revision Deletion Editorial	Page	Code	Page	Addition Revision Deletion Editorial	Page
D7858	67			D7962	71	Addition	98
D7860	68			D7963	71		
D7865	68			D7970	71		
D7870	68			D7971	71		
D7871	68			D7972	71		
D7872	68			D7979	71		
D7873	68			D7980	71		
D7874	68			D7981	71		
D7875	68			D7982	71		
D7876	68			D7983	71		
D7877	68			D7990	72		
D7880	68			D7991	72		
D7881	68			D7993	72	Addition	98
D7899	68			D7994	72	Addition	98
D7910	69			D7995	72		
D7911	69			D7996	72		
D7912	69			D7997	72		
D7920	69			D7998	72		
D7921	69			D7999	72		
D7922	69			XI. Orthodontics			
D7940	69			D8010	73		
D7941	69			D8020	73		
D7943	69			D8030	73		
D7944	69			D8040	73		
D7945	69			D8050	74		
D7946	69			D8060	74		
D7947	70			D8070	74		
D7948	70			D8080	74		
D7949	70			D8090	74		
D7950	70			D8210	75		
D7951	70			D8220	75		
D7952	70			D8660	75		
D7953	70			D8670	75		
D7955	71			D8680	75		
~~D7960~~		Deletion		D8681	75		
D7961	71	Addition	98	D8690	75		

CDT Category		Code Entry Change (when applicable)			CDT Category		Code Entry Change (when applicable)	
Code	Page	Addition Revision Deletion Editorial	Page		Code	Page	Addition Revision Deletion Editorial	Page
D8695	75				D9910	80		
D8696	75				D9911	80		
D8697	75				D9920	80		
D8698	75				D9930	81		
D8699	75				D9932	81		
D8701	76				D9933	81		
D8702	76				D9934	81		
D8703	76				D9935	81		
D8704	76				D9941	81		
D8999	76				D9942	81		
XII. Adjunctive General Services					D9943	81		
D9110	77				D9944	81		
D9120	77				D9945	81		
D9130	77				D9946	81		
D9210	77				D9950	81		
D9211	77				D9951	82		
D9212	77				D9952	82		
D9215	77				D9961	82		
D9219	77				D9970	82		
D9222	78				D9971	82	Revision	100
D9223	78				D9972	82		
D9230	78				D9973	82		
D9239	78				D9974	82		
D9243	78				D9975	82		
D9248	78				D9985	82		
D9310	79				D9986	82		
D9311	79				D9987	82		
D9410	79				D9990	83		
D9420	79				D9991	83		
D9430	79				D9992	83		
D9440	79				D9993	83		
D9450	79				D9994	83		
D9610	80				D9995	83		
D9612	80				D9996	84		
D9613	80				D9997	83		
D9630	80				D9999	84		

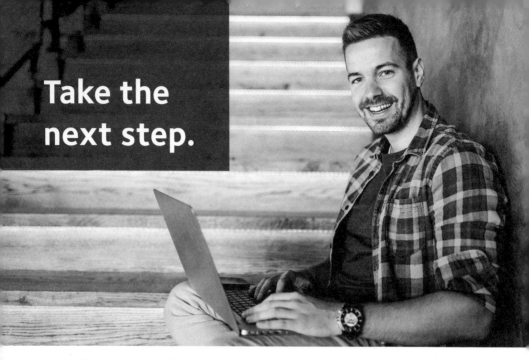

Take the next step.

You have the codes, now learn how to use them in practice.

Mastery of the CDT codes will make you a more valuable asset to the team and practice. Increase your coding skills and complete the **ADA Dental Coding Certificate: Assessment-Based CDT Course**. It helps new and experienced staff members achieve coding proficiency and help the dental office run more smoothly.

Participants will:

- Gain thorough knowledge of coding terms and tools
- Understand dental procedure codes and how to apply them
- Accurately complete the ADA Dental Claim Form
- Use the *CDT* and *CDT Companion* books correctly

As the official source for CDT® codes, the ADA has answered thousands of questions over the years. When dental teams have questions, we have the answers. Take advantage of our expertise and get up to code today!

After successfully passing the online assessment, **participants will earn 4 CE hours**. The course is available either with or without CDT books.

> **Save 20%** on this essential course and train your staff with promo code **CDTTeam2021** by 5.28.2021. Register today at **ADACEOnline.org**.